The Medicine Show

The Medicine Show

Consumers Union's
practical guide to some
everyday health problems
and health products

by the Editors of Consumer Reports
Consumers Union, Mount Vernon, New York

THE MEDICINE SHOW is a special publication of Consumers Union, the nonprofit organization that publishes CONSUMER REPORTS, the monthly magazine of test reports, product Ratings, and buying guidance. Established in 1936, Consumers Union is chartered under the Not-For-Profit Corporation Law of the State of New York.

The purposes of Consumers Union, as stated in its charter, are to provide consumers with information and counsel on consumer goods and services, to give information and assistance on all matters relating to the expenditure of the family income, and to initiate and to cooperate with individual and group efforts seeking to create and maintain decent living standards.

Consumers Union derives its income solely from the sale of CONSUMER REPORTS (magazine and TV) and other publications. CU accepts no advertising or product samples, and is not beholden in any way to any commercial interest. Its Ratings and reports are solely for the information and use of the readers of its publications.

Neither the Ratings nor the reports, including this book, may be used in advertising or for any commercial purpose. Consumers Union will take all steps open to it to prevent or to prosecute any such uses of its material, its name, or the name of CONSUMER REPORTS.

Preface

THIS EDITION of THE MEDICINE SHOW, like earlier editions, is based on articles originally published in the pages of CONSUMER REPORTS, the monthly magazine of Consumers Union. All such material has been extensively reworked, updated, and expanded. Some chapters contained in previous editions have been dropped, and several new chapters have been included. Consumers Union has had the expert advice and technical assistance of many consultants who helped develop and revise all this material.

Chief among the consultants and principally responsible for the contents of THE MEDICINE SHOW are Consumers Union's two medical advisers, Marvin M. Lipman, M.D., and Harold Aaron, M.D. Dr. Lipman has been medical adviser of Consumers Union since 1967. He is a diplomate of the American Board of Internal Medicine, certified in endocrinology and metabolism, a fellow of the American College of Physicians, a member of the American Federation for Clinical Research, and Clinical Associate Professor of Medicine at New York Medical College. Dr. Aaron has been medical adviser of Consumers Union since its founding in 1936. He is a diplomate of the American Board of Internal Medicine, and a fellow of the New York Academy of Medicine, of the New York Academy of Sciences, and of the American Public Health Association. He is also chairman of the editorial board of *The Medical Letter* (see below).

A number of respected books and periodicals were consulted in the preparation of THE MEDICINE SHOW. Basic sources, frequently cited in this edition, included: *The Pharmacological Basis of Therapeutics*, a pharmacology, toxicology, and therapeutics text for physicians and medical students, edited by Drs. Louis S. Goodman and Alfred Gilman, fourth edition, published by Macmillan; *AMA Drug Evaluations*, second edition, published by the Department of Drugs, American Medical Association; *Handbook of Non-Prescription Drugs*, fourth edition, published by the American Pharmaceutical Association; and *The Medical Letter*, a nonprofit periodical for medical professionals containing evaluations of medicinal drugs in terms of effectiveness, safety, and possible alternatives.

THE MEDICINE SHOW includes frequent references to products by brand name, usually in discussions of specific products. Often, in general discussions, brand names — particularly of drugs, both prescription and those purchased over the counter (OTC) — are mentioned as examples and for ease of identification. Such references are not intended as a comprehensive listing of all brands available.

In the text, the brand names of OTC drugs are capitalized and italicized. The brand names of prescription drugs are capitalized; representative brand names often appear in parentheses immediately following the generic name of a prescription drug. For example, a widely prescribed anticoagulant is referred to in the text as "warfarin (Athrombin-K, Coumadin, Panwarfin)"; warfarin is the drug's generic name, while the three products named are some of the brands of warfarin available.

To supplement the general index, which starts on page 375, a second index — of brand-name products — has been added to THE MEDICINE SHOW. Beginning on page 370, this product index lists the brand names of all drugs (both OTC and prescription), cosmetics, and medical devices mentioned in the book.

This edition of THE MEDICINE SHOW also includes, beginning on page 348, a glossary of select words and phrases appearing in the book. We urge readers to use the glossary for a better understanding not only of THE MEDICINE SHOW but of medical language encountered elsewhere.

Contents

Introduction

MANY "EVERYDAY HEALTH PROBLEMS" are more annoying than dangerous, more a bother than a threat. Left to their own devices, most people would be quite capable of coping with such problems. But people are not let alone. Indeed, they are all but overwhelmed by expressions of concern and advice — from television and radio commercials, advertisements in newspapers and magazines, "news" stories of miraculous medical discoveries, and label claims on the products filling the shelves of drugstores and supermarkets. Their peace and their wallets are threatened — and sometimes their health.

It is truly a medicine show. No one questions the energy, the ingenuity, or the skill of its promoters. Not all are crude hawkers of snake oil; some of the sales pitches are positively low-keyed. What thoughtful consumers should challenge is the extent to which the hucksters succeed in becoming the medical educators of the buyers. The education takes a predictable form. Virtually all promoters of health products proceed in the same pattern — inducing alarm so that they can offer reassurance, and then promising benefit with every bottle, jar, and tube. And since selling is their prime purpose, they state no more than what is in their interest.

But huckstering should not be confused with education, particularly education on matters of health and medicine. Over the years more and more consumers have come to question the reliability of drug advertising. They have learned that, despite the warnings and the promises, the contents of the bottles, jars, and tubes are often less than represented and sometimes downright worthless. Some are even harmful.

Reliable information on health and medicine is needed, and Consumers Union looks to the time when responsible drug advertising will better meet that need. Meanwhile, this book offers consumers "a restorative of balance and perspective, an antidote to excesses, and a purgative for much nonsense" (as stated in 1961 in the first edition of THE MEDICINE SHOW).

Now thoroughly revised and brought up to date, this latest edition of THE MEDICINE SHOW is intended to help consumers better understand the differences between genuine advances in health and medicine and the exaggerated claims of the sellers.

The ailments do not change much from year to year, and neither do the remedies. Old familiar "miracles" of drug advertising still burst upon the scene, only to fade away and be replaced by new ones. Regulations catch up with deceptions. New fads replace old ones. Fresh claims are cranked out to beguile the consumer.

Unfortunately, many people continue to believe such claims. In 1972 the Food and Drug Administration released a study of American health practices and opinions. Those surveyed were presented with the statement that advertisements about medications and health aids "must be true or they wouldn't be allowed to say them." *Thirty-eight percent of those surveyed — representing fifty million Americans eighteen and over — agreed with the statement.*

But not all consumers are "believers"; many still refuse to accept the hucksters' medicine show at face value. Like Consumers Union, they question the propriety and the quality of drug advertising as a source of information about health and medicine. This new edition of THE MEDICINE SHOW, like the earlier ones, is addressed not only to these skeptics and truth-seekers, but also to those who may still be susceptible to the blandishments of the hucksters.

THE MEDICINE SHOW seeks to help consumers make better choices — when choices are available — in many areas of health and medicine. For example, the book offers some insights into the puzzling world of prescription drugs, where the pharmaceutical company provides, the physician prescribes, the pharmacist fulfills, and the patient — the consumer — pays and has little or no say.

The thinking of many physicians and of other consultants to Consumers Union is represented here, and doctors should find the book a useful adjunct to their efforts to give their patients sound guidance in medical matters. But THE MEDICINE SHOW is not primarily for doctors, nor even for patients. It is above all for consumers who want a source of health information significantly more reliable than the next television commercial.

Chapter 1

Aspirin
and
its competitors

ASPIRIN, IN ALL ITS VARIOUS DISGUISES, is the most common of
all over-the-counter (OTC) medications. It can be bought
plain or buffered, in effervescent tablets or powders, alone or
in combination with other analgesics, antacids, antihistamines,
and decongestants, and in countless "special" remedies highly
touted for arthritis and rheumatism. Soon aspirin may be available in liquid form, too. Sales of analgesic products already run
more than $700 million a year — an amount exceeded only by
that spent for OTC cold and cough items.

Although the number and quantity of inert ingredients used
in the formulation and manufacture of aspirin tablets may vary
among pharmaceutical companies, for most people the only
practical difference among standard 5-grain brands of aspirin
tablets, plain or buffered, is price. *Any* brand of this widely
used drug can be an effective remedy for symptomatic relief
as an antipyretic and an analgesic in a variety of common ailments. It reduces fever and aches in common respiratory infections such as colds, grippe, and flu, and relieves tension
headaches and joint and muscle aches, as well as mild menstrual
cramps. For some people it even works as a mild sedative.
And, in many patients with chronic rheumatoid arthritis, it
seems nearly as effective in reducing inflammation and swelling

of joints as cortisone or its steroid analogues — and is far safer. Aspirin is also a mainstay in the treatment of the more common osteoarthritis. (See Chapter 19 for a discussion of aspirin products specially promoted for arthritis.)

On the debit side, too, all aspirin is pretty much the same. Really severe pain, such as that experienced by migraine sufferers, is usually not relieved by this drug, either alone or in combination with other OTC analgesic agents. A few people are truly allergic to aspirin and may react with hives or asthma. Such allergic persons should, of course, avoid aspirin in any form or combination (see page 20). Some people may find that aspirin upsets the stomach, particularly when used frequently or in large doses.

Chronic use of aspirin or products containing aspirin, most likely because of the irritative effect on the stomach lining, may lead to iron-deficiency anemia. This anemia is due to daily loss, over a long period of time, of small amounts of blood — too small to be discernible — in the stool. There is some evidence that the use of buffered aspirin minimizes this side effect. Enteric-coated aspirin (such as *A.S.A. Enseals* and *Ecotrin*) has a specially formulated outer coating which retards disintegration in the stomach, thereby lessening the chance of such irritation. The product is not foolproof, however; on occasion, whole tablets may be found in the stool. Long-term users of aspirin products require periodic blood counts (every few months) so that their physicians can determine the need for possible iron replacement.

One form of aspirin — chewing gum — is not recommended by CU's medical consultants. *Aspergum* is widely advertised "for minor sore throat pain"; yet aspirin is devoid of any topical anesthetic action. Any benefit derived from this type of preparation can come only from its absorption into the bloodstream from the intestinal tract once the saliva/aspirin mixture is swallowed. One piece of *Aspergum* contains about two-thirds of the aspirin content in the usual 5-grain tablet. It would be more effective (and cheaper) to swallow a 5-grain aspirin tablet — and then, if you must, to chew a piece of "sugarless" gum. CU's medical consultants say it is far more effective for relief of sore throat discomfort to stick to the traditional remedy: gargling with warm salt water (see Chapter 4). Gargling with crushed aspirin in water is not only ineffective for the relief of a sore throat, but aspirin particles may actually cause injury if they are not swallowed and remain in contact with the delicate membranes of an inflamed throat.

Pharmacies and other retail stores often sell unadvertised or "house" brands of aspirin at retail prices ranging from 17¢ to 59¢ per hundred. (CU knows of no reason to buy anything but the least expensive brand.) To command a higher price some manufacturers add one or more ingredients and several million dollars worth of advertising to convince the public that they offer something better than plain old aspirin.

In fact, in March 1973 the Federal Trade Commission (FTC) issued orders to three manufacturers of ten leading analgesic products and to their five advertising agencies to halt what the FTC alleged were misleading advertising claims. However, Glenbrook (the makers of *Bayer Aspirin, Bayer Children's Aspirin, Cope, Midol,* and *Vanquish*), Bristol-Meyers (the makers of *Bufferin, Excedrin,* and *Excedrin P.M.*), and Whitehall (the makers of *Anacin* and *Arthritis Pain Formula*) denied the allegations and called unconstitutional the FTC proposal that the manufacturers be compelled to correct any misrepresentations.

After examining the documents submitted by the makers of *Bufferin*, the FTC found no reasonable basis for the claim that *Bufferin* works "twice as fast as aspirin." Buffered aspirin, which includes small amounts of antacid, has been shown to be somewhat more rapidly absorbed into the bloodstream than unbuffered aspirin. *Bufferin's* maker exploited these tests as substantiation for its claim. But in 1971 the Panel on Drugs for Relief of Pain of the National Academy of Sciences–National Research Council (NAS–NRC) called that claim "ambiguous and misleading." While recognizing the possibility of slightly faster absorption, the panel concluded that "there is no evidence to indicate that the speed of onset of analgesic action is significantly increased." Furthermore, a recent study demonstrated that generic buffered aspirin — much less expensive than *Bufferin* — dissolves as fast as the name brand.

Bufferin claims that it "helps prevent the stomach upset often caused by aspirin," ostensibly because it includes, besides the usual amount of aspirin, very small amounts of two common antacids. The NAS–NRC panel reported that most studies it evaluated showed "little difference in the incidence or intensity of subjective gastrointestinal side effects after ingestion of *Bufferin* or plain aspirin."

The panel, in short, found no convincing support for claims that *Bufferin* is either "faster" or "gentler" than straight aspirin. (*Arthritis Strength Bufferin* is like *Bufferin*, except that it contains 50 percent more aspirin per tablet and slightly more of the antacids — see table on page 22.)

"Combination analgesic products appear to have no clinical advantage over single component products," advises the American Pharmaceutical Association's *Handbook of Non-Prescription Drugs.* "These combinations, for the most part, are of greater economic significance to the manufacturer than increased therapeutic benefit to the patient." Through constant and often misleading advertising, such manufacturers now get the lion's share of what consumers spend on pain relievers.

Those in pain have been persuaded to buy "shotgun" remedies containing many ingredients — apparently on the theory that if they use enough ingredients, at least one might work. A combination of aspirin, phenacetin, and caffeine, known as the *A.P.C.* tablet, has enjoyed considerable popularity. *Anacin* entered its initial bid for the aspirin jackpot by formulating a similar shotgun preparation containing aspirin, acetanilid, and caffeine. The ads announced that *Anacin* is "like a doctor's prescription," containing not just one or two but *three* ingredients. When acetanilid was shown to cause certain blood disturbances, *Anacin* substituted phenacetin. When development of kidney problems was linked with phenacetin (a linkage still under dispute among authorities), phenacetin too was dropped.

Citing the growing evidence of a relationship between kidney damage and phenacetin in combination drugs, in June 1973 Canada forbade the marketing of all medications containing phenacetin in combination with any salt or derivative of acetylsalicylic acid (aspirin). Since 1964 the Food and Drug Administration has taken note of the hazards of phenacetin by requiring a warning on labels of all preparations containing the drug. CU's medical consultants urge consumers to avoid analgesic combinations that include phenacetin in their formulation (see table on page 22).

With phenacetin dropped from the formulation, the *Anacin* sold currently contains only aspirin and caffeine. The amount of caffeine in an *Anacin* tablet is about as much as that in a quarter cup of brewed coffee. There is no evidence, declares *AMA Drug Evaluations* in a discussion of these *A.P.C.* preparations, that such a small dose of caffeine "has an analgesic effect or that it affects the activity of the analgesic components." Thus the only effective analgesic in *Anacin* is aspirin, the anonymous "pain-reliever doctors recommend most for headaches," according to the *Anacin* ads — which are under attack by the FTC.

An *Anacin* tablet contains 6.17 grains of aspirin instead of the usual 5 grains. A recent price survey indicated that a tablet of *Anacin* sells at more than four times the price of a 5-grain tablet of ordinary low-cost aspirin. This is a high premium to pay for an additional 1.17 grains of aspirin per tablet plus the amount of caffeine in a quarter cup of coffee. (The makers of *Anacin* also market *Arthritis Pain Formula* analgesic tablets; each tablet contains 7.5 grains of aspirin.)

If three ingredients are good, four must be better — at least from an advertising standpoint. So enter *Excedrin* — another target of FTC charges of misleading advertising claims.

One of *Excedrin's* ingredients is aspirin — 3 grains of it. Another is acetaminophen (about 1.5 grains), an analgesic roughly comparable to aspirin for relieving pain and fever. Acetaminophen's advantage is as an alternative drug for those allergic to aspirin or for others who should not take aspirin for any of several reasons (see page 20). There is no such advantage when acetaminophen is combined with aspirin in *Excedrin* or other shotgun preparations. *Excedrin's* third ingredient is 2 grains of salicylamide. *AMA Drug Evaluations* reports that salicylamide "is much less effective than aspirin" for pain or fever when given in the same dose, and that it is "too weak and unreliable to be useful."

Finally, one *Excedrin* contains 65 milligrams of caffeine, twice as much as *Anacin* or *Bromo Seltzer*. So those who take eight *Excedrin* tablets in a day — the maximum recommended on the label — are getting 520 milligrams of caffeine, or the equivalent of four cups of coffee. Thus it is not surprising that some people who take the maximum daily dosage of *Excedrin* — on top of their usual caffeine intake in coffee, tea, and cola drinks — may become jittery.

On the basis of *Excedrin's* formula, CU wonders how it can be called an "extra-strength pain reliever." It contains about 4.5 grains of effective analgesics — aspirin and acetaminophen — plus 3 grains of dubious or ineffective ingredients: salicylamide and caffeine. "Judging from the formula," says Dr. Richard P. Penna of the American Pharmaceutical Association, "You would have to conclude the drug is no more effective than 5 grains of aspirin." (*Excedrin P.M.* is like *Excedrin* — see table on page 22 — except that the caffeine is supplanted by a small amount of methapyrilene — an antihistamine which has a mildly sedative effect.)

Vanquish and *Cope*, touted as "new" OTC analgesics, are merely further variations on the same familiar theme — but each has *five* ingredients. Like *Excedrin*, *Vanquish* contains aspirin, acetaminophen, and caffeine; and like *Bufferin*, it includes small amounts of two antacids. *Cope* also contains aspirin and caffeine, plus the same two antacids as *Vanquish*. *Cope's* fifth ingredient is methapyrilene, the same antihistamine found in *Excedrin P.M.* And like *Excedrin* and *Bufferin*, *Vanquish* and *Cope* are also the targets of FTC charges of misleading advertising.

Many drugs are greeted with great enthusiasm when first marketed; subsequent experience tempers the initial glow. But aspirin is different. Well-controlled studies suggest that it is even more effective than was formerly supposed.

A Mayo Clinic study published in 1972, for example, compared plain aspirin not only with acetaminophen and phenacetin, but also with a range of allegedly more potent and far more expensive pain relievers available only on prescription — including codeine, propoxyphene (Darvon), ethoheptazine (Zactane), and mefenamic acid (Ponstel). Each drug was given orally, in random order. The dosage for each was the recognized therapeutic equivalent of that for the other drugs, and all were enclosed in identical blue capsules. Some capsules were placebos. The tests were double-blind; that is, neither physicians nor patients knew what the capsules contained until the results were recorded. The fifty-seven patients in the study all suffered from pain judged to be mild to moderate, occurring in various parts of the body and associated with inoperable cancer.

The results can be summarized briefly. No drug in the study had a significantly faster onset of relief than aspirin or a significantly longer duration of relief than aspirin. The number of side effects reported for aspirin did not differ significantly from the number reported for the placebo. Aspirin led the list when it came to the proportion of patients experiencing at least 50 percent relief of pain. The average estimated percentage of pain relieved was higher for aspirin than for any of the other drugs.

The investigators concluded: "In this study, simple aspirin at a dosage of 650 milligrams [equivalent to two 5-grain tablets] was the superior agent for relief of cancer pain among the tested marketed analgesics. Indeed, among all analgesics and narcotics available for oral use, none have been demonstrated to show a consistent advantage over aspirin for the relief of any type of pain."

An interesting but not unexpected sidelight of the study was the response of patients to the placebo. Twenty-one percent claimed greater than 50 percent relief of pain with the dummy medication. Such a result, which is common in medical experience, is called the placebo effect. In essence, those who believe a certain medication will help them, obtain relief from it even if it has no pharmacological effect. The same principle often applies to OTC remedies, and sometimes explains why one drug seems to work while a virtually identical one does not.

Moreover, Darvon, one of the expensive prescription analgesics used in the Mayo Clinic study, had already been shown in an earlier study published in the *Journal of the American Medical Association* to be no more and perhaps less effective than aspirin. The authors of the report noted, "The fact that a drug is sold by prescription in no way proves its efficacy and potency." They concluded: "Our review prompts us to recommend aspirin as the mild analgesic of choice. If aspirin does not provide adequate relief, it is unlikely that Darvon will do so."

For people who are allergic to aspirin, have stomach disorders, gout, or are taking anticoagulants, CU's medical consultants recommend acetaminophen. (Some people are allergic to acetaminophen, but toxicity has been reported only in cases of massive overdosage.) Most studies indicate that acetaminophen is roughly comparable to aspirin in similar doses for temporary relief of pains and aches and for lowering fever. Because it lacks aspirin's effect on inflammation, however, it cannot replace aspirin in the overall treatment of connective tissue diseases such as rheumatoid arthritis or acute rheumatic fever.

Acetaminophen is available in tablets, and in liquid form or as drops for infants and others who are unable to take tablets. It can be purchased without a prescription under its generic name and under ten or more brand names — such as *Liquiprin* (for children), *Tempra*, *Tylenol*, and *Valadol*. As in the case of aspirin, CU recommends whichever is cheapest. The dosage schedule is identical to that for aspirin (see below).

Although *Alka-Seltzer* is widely advertised as an antacid for digestive disturbances, CU's medical consultants advise against its regular use for that purpose because its aspirin content makes it unsuitable as a digestive aid (see Chapter 7). As a pain reliever, though, *Alka-Seltzer* has some merit. It must be dissolved in a glass of water before it can be taken, which reduces its time in the stomach, hence minimizing possible gastric irritation. However, it contains so much bicarbonate that it should *not* be taken daily over long periods. And its sodium content is so high that it should not be used *at all* by anyone on a low-salt diet. Those tempted by the ads to depend on *Alka-Seltzer* for regular relief from the simultaneous discomfort of headache and upset stomach should take particular note of these warnings against the frequent use of *Alka-Seltzer*.

An *Alka-Seltzer* tablet contains 5 grains of aspirin. For relief of mild to moderate pain, two *Alka-Seltzer* tablets, therefore, are the equivalent of two aspirin tablets. The cost, of course, is substantially higher. Because of its high price and sodium bicarbonate content, CU's medical consultants do not recommend *Alka-Seltzer* (or a similar product such as *Fizrin*) over plain aspirin taken with a full glass of water. However, for a person

Ingredients of some analgesic products

All ingredients in this table are listed in grains per tablet.*

	Aspirin	Other analgesics
Alka-Seltzer†	5.00	—
Anacin	6.17	—
A.P.C.	3.49	phenacetin, 2.50
Arthritis Pain Formula	7.50	—
Arthritis Strength Bufferin	7.50	—
Bayer Aspirin	5.00	—
Bayer Timed-Release Aspirin	10.00	—
Bufferin	5.00	—
Cope	6.50	—
Ecotrin	4.63	—
Empirin Compound	3.50	phenacetin, 2.50
Excedrin	3.00	acetaminophen, 1.50; salicylamide, 2.00
Excedrin P.M.	3.00	acetaminophen, 2.50; salicylamide, 2.00
Vanquish	3.50	acetaminophen, 3.00

* Labels on analgesic products also give some ingredients in milligrams; 1 grain = 64.8 milligrams.

† Also contains citric acid (16.28 grains) and monocalcium phosphate (3 grains).

Caffeine	Antihistamine	Antacid
—	—	sodium bicarbonate, 29.38
0.50	—	—
0.50	—	—
—	—	dried aluminum hydroxide gel; magnesium hydroxide‡
—	—	aluminum glycinate, 1.13; magnesium carbonate, 2.25
—	—	—
—	—	—
—	—	aluminum glycinate, 0.75; magnesium carbonate, 1.50
0.50	methapyrilene, 0.19	dried aluminum hydroxide gel, 0.39; magnesium hydroxide, 0.77
—	—	—
0.50	—	—
1.00	—	—
—	methapyrilene, 0.39	—
0.51	—	dried aluminum hydroxide gel, 0.39; magnesium hydroxide, 0.77

‡ Quantities not available from manufacturer.

Sources: Product label; product manufacturer; *Handbook of Non-Prescription Drugs*, 1973 Edition, American Pharmaceutical Association; *Physicians' Desk Reference*, 27th Edition, 1973, Medical Economics Co.

who experiences mild stomach distress even when aspirin is taken with the recommended quantity of water, the occasional use of a soluble form of aspirin seems reasonable.

Aspirin's caveats are important:

■ Prolonged use of aspirin for chronic conditions, such as rheumatoid arthritis, should be monitored by a physician.

■ Drink a full glass of water or other liquid with your aspirin to minimize possible stomach irritation.

■ Unless instructed to do so by your physician, do not take more than 10 to 15 grains (two or three tablets) at a time, do not take aspirin more often than every four hours, and do not take more than ten tablets in twenty-four hours. One of the earliest symptoms of chronic aspirin overdosage is ringing in the ears, sometimes accompanied by a decrease in hearing ability. These effects are reversible when the dosage is lowered.

■ Some people are sensitive or allergic to aspirin. If you are among them, acetaminophen is a reasonable alternative. Since many combination OTC products contain aspirin, be sure to read labels.

■ Some people experience mild stomach distress when they take aspirin. If you are among them, consider acetaminophen or a soluble form of aspirin, which can be dissolved in a glass of water before you take it.

■ Patients with a history of stomach ulcers or gout as well as those on oral antidiabetic medications should consult a physician before taking aspirin.

■ Aspirin retards blood clotting in several ways. Hence patients with bleeding disorders and patients using anticoagulants such as warfarin (Athrombin-K, Coumadin, Panwarfin) should take aspirin sparingly, if at all. There is also some evidence that pregnant women (see Chapter 23) approaching term or patients about to undergo elective surgery should not take aspirin one to two weeks before they are scheduled for hospitalization.

Pregnant women should also avoid taking aspirin for the week or two prior to term because of possibly affecting the blood-clotting mechanism of the newborn. Among those taking high dosages of aspirin there is some evidence of added risk of prolonged labor and an increase in the average duration of pregnancy.

■ For children's doses, consult the label. Usually, each dose for a child should not exceed 1 grain per year of age (up to a maximum of 5 grains). Children can be given the recommended dose crushed in a little applesauce, jelly, or honey if they dislike taking it straight. If children prefer to take their aspirin adult-style, be sure they drink a full glass of liquid along with it. If

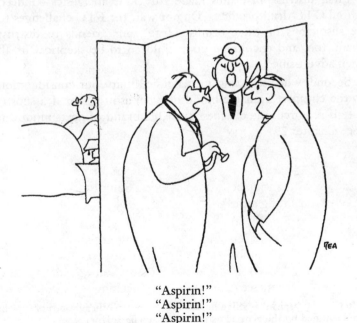

"Aspirin!"
"Aspirin!"
"Aspirin!"

you buy flavored aspirin, remember that it can be mistaken for candy.

■ *Keep aspirin and other drugs out of reach of children.* In 1974, the latest year for which statistics are available, twenty-four children less than five years of age died after ingesting overdoses of aspirin or other salicylates. This total accounted for about 18 percent of all accidental deaths from poisoning among children in that age group.

■ The use of so-called timed-release aspirin preparations is not advised. As with so many of these products, absorption may be irregular and adverse reactions prolonged (see page 36).

Finally, CU's medical consultants have two basic recommendations:

First, distrust all claims made for OTC analgesics — indeed for all OTC drug products. Do not wait for FTC challenges to be suspicious of these claims. Urge your friends to distrust them, too, and encourage your children to be skeptical of all such advertising.

Second, when selecting an analgesic, limit your consideration to the cheapest available brand of plain aspirin,* or if a substitute is required, the cheapest available brand of acetaminophen (see Chapter 29).

---

* In Canada "aspirin" is still a Bayer trade name, so other brands of aspirin are identified by the generic name acetylsalicylic acid, or ASA.

Chapter 2

The common cold

ALTHOUGH THE PAST FIFTY YEARS have seen more medical progress than any other period in history, and although the common cold has been estimated to cost almost $5 billion each year in lost wages and medical expenses, no means has yet been found to prevent or cure it.

In fact, the common cold, known in medical jargon as the "coryza" syndrome, is not a simple matter; rather, it is a complex of symptoms. Caused by any one of a group of viruses (currently estimated at about 100 in number), the common cold is primarily an infection of the lining membrane of the upper respiratory tract, including the nose, the sinuses, and the throat. This delicate membrane reacts to infection by swelling and by increasing the rate of mucus formation, leading to congestion, stuffiness, and probably a good deal of nose blowing. Due to loss of the nasal cavity as a resonating chamber, a characteristic change in voice quality also occurs. The increased mucus flow usually causes postnasal drip, which is irritating and contributes to the familiar "scratchy" throat and cough.

The sinuses, which normally empty into the nasal cavity, may become blocked by excessive swelling of the membranes. The resultant increase in sinus pressure may cause a frontal headache. In similar fashion, swelling in the upper part of the throat can block the Eustachian tubes — the two narrow canals that lead to the ears. This blockage can cause accumulation of fluid and pressure in the middle ear, which may be painful. Less commonly, an unpleasant spinning sensation known as vertigo may result.

A cold is usually self-limited, lasting about one to two weeks. At any time during the course of a cold, bacteria (such as staphylococci or pneumococci) can be secondary invaders, bringing on debilitating infections of the sinuses and ears. However, the old warning that, if you don't take care, a cold will turn into pneumonia, is hardly ever true. Pneumonia and most other infections of the lower respiratory tract begin in the bronchi and the lungs rather than in the upper respiratory tract.

Fever above 101°F on a rectal thermometer is not usually part of an uncomplicated cold. Although mild elevation of temperature can occur, most people stay home from work or school because of generalized symptoms — muscle ache, weakness, and fatigue. The extent of these symptoms varies with the individual. If fever above 101°F rectally persists beyond two days, medical advice should be sought.

Americans spend $735 million a year for cold and cough remedies. Advertisers have claimed preventive and curative virtues for vitamins, alkalizers, lemon drinks, antihistamines, decongestants, timed-release capsules, antibiotics, antiseptic gargles, bioflavonoids, nose drops and sprays, quinine pills, aspirin mixtures, laxatives, inhalers, aromatic salves, liniments, room air sprays, and a variety of other products. Many of these drugs do neither good nor harm to the cold victim; but there is no doubt that they benefit the drug manufacturers.

Everyone has heard of sure-fire formulas for preventing a cold. Popular home methods include daily cold showers, regular exercise, and drinking lots of water. Some people swear by cod-liver oil, alcoholic beverages, citrus fruit juices (or massive doses of vitamin C), or keeping one's feet dry. At one time, many industrial establishments encouraged their employees to submit to inoculations with cold "vaccines." And splendid results from these programs were regularly reported. But such vaccines, like many other "scientific" (or folk) remedies, have gradually been abandoned as experience and controlled testing have proved their uselessness in preventing colds. This year, just as fifty years ago, Americans on the average will suffer two to three colds a year, the acute infectious stages of which will last about a week or two (although a cough or postnasal drip may linger), regardless of any physical measure, diet, or drug used to try to head them off.

It is most unfortunate that the name "cold" has been given to this common, but minor, malady. The name has led many people to infer — incorrectly — that the common cold is somehow caused by a drop in the environmental temperature. There is as yet no evidence that the common cold ever occurs in the absence of an infecting organism. Moreover, studies have shown that chilling does not predispose one to infection with the cold virus (or viruses). The increased incidence of colds in winter probably reflects the fact that much time is spent indoors, thereby facilitating the transfer of viruses from person to person. In fact, one is less likely to catch a cold after a solitary walk, barefoot in a rainstorm, than after mixing with a convivial group of snifflers and sneezers at a fireside gathering.

The common cold, it is now reasonably certain, is spread not so much by sneezing and coughing — or even kissing — as by shaking hands and handling contaminated matter. The home, office, classroom, bus, or any other place where people gather is a good spreading ground. But resistance seems to vary greatly among individuals, so that not everyone exposed to a common source of infection becomes ill. Moreover, the natural factors — whatever they are — that contribute to resistance in an individual may be operative at one time and not at another. Thus it is not uncommon for some unlucky person to have a "bad year," suffering from as many as five or six colds, and then remain in excellent health during the following year or two. These variations in host resistance and the irregular pattern in the occurrence of colds help make it extremely difficult to evaluate cold medications.

This has not stopped the manufacturers of cold preparations from palming off on an all-too-willing public a series of gimmicks and "cure-alls" for the prevention or treatment of cold symptoms.

Because one way in which colds are transmitted is by small moisture droplets in the air, attempts have been made to sterilize the air — with special ultraviolet lamps, with sprays of such chemicals as triethylene glycol, or with air purifiers containing "germicidal filters" or producing negative ions. These approaches have not been successful.

The most recent development in this category is aerosol medication.* The product releases a spray compounded of menthol (an organic alcohol with a medicinal scent), glycols (antibacterial agents long ago shown to be without therapeutic value when sprayed in the air), and flavoring oils. Even if the ingredients were effective, common sense should make one wonder how a large enough dose could be delivered when the product is so widely dispersed in the air. Furthermore, CU's medical consultants do not know of any published reports of controlled trials supporting the claim that these preparations can relieve congestion.

After the death of a five-year-old girl who had been exposed to *Pertussin Night-Time Medicated Vaporizer Spray*, the Food and Drug Administration (FDA) in July 1973 ordered the recall of that preparation and later reported that twenty-one deaths since 1968 had been associated with its use. The FDA

---

* For a warning about the possible hazards of using aerosol spray products in the home, see page 311.

attributed the spray's toxicity to the presence of trichloroethane, an organic solvent. Five additional brands having the same chemical solvent as an ingredient in the spray were also recalled by the FDA. As of this writing, the FDA is investigating all over-the-counter (OTC) decongestant aerosol sprays to assess their safety.

On another front, attempts to increase natural resistance to colds by modifying the diet have also failed. Most medical scientists now agree that until an antiviral drug is developed, or until a reliable vaccine is perfected, no real progress in limiting the spread or incidence of colds can be anticipated.

But if colds cannot be prevented, can't the symptoms at least be checked or relieved? Here, too, there are determined advocates of a wide variety of home remedies and equally determined supporters of the large number of OTC products. Much research on cold remedies is scientifically worthless because of the difficulty in making an accurate diagnosis of the common cold. One reason is that the term "cold" may designate not only identifiable viral respiratory infections, but also almost any congestion of the nose, caused by a variety of irritants, including smog, or by allergens. Such noninfectious congestion may last a few minutes, several hours, or even days. Any medication, even a sugar pill, may seem to be remarkably effective if the congestion is of short duration. Studies have also failed because they did not allow for the unpredictable course of colds and their varying incidence. The effect of the emotions on cold symptoms is also a factor.

Antihistamines provide a case in point. Their popularity in cold treatment began with an enthusiastic clinical study by a physician who, impressed by the effect of antihistamines on hay fever (an allergy), tried them on people with colds and found them helpful in shortening the colds or controlling the symptoms. Other doctors, impressed by the first report, tried antihistamines with their patients and reported equally favorable results in treating the common cold.

But physicians who are expert in diagnosis and treatment of sickness may not be equally knowledgeable in the evaluation of clinical drug trials (see Chapter 26). Rigid criteria must be met to prove the efficacy of an agent claimed to prevent, treat, or abort a disease. When clinicians properly investigated the effect of antihistamines on the common cold, they found that a placebo gave results just as good as those from the much-hailed drug. In short, antihistamines have proved of no value against the common cold; furthermore, they produce in many users such side effects as drowsiness, dizziness, and headache.

The pitch for bioflavonoids for relief of colds came after the disillusionment with antihistamines. Bioflavonoids, a group of complex organic substances, are collectively called vitamin P and believed, although never proved, to have a strengthening effect on the capillary blood vessels. That bioflavonoids were as disappointing as antihistamines in the treatment of colds has also been amply demonstrated. In 1968 the FDA determined from its findings and those of the National Academy of Sciences–National Research Council that flavonoid drugs, including bioflavonoids, were not effective "for use in man for any condition." Remedies containing bioflavonoids are no longer widely marketed.

The next fad in the hotly competitive cold remedy field was the introduction of products for oral use containing several ingredients in fixed combinations. (*Contac, Dristan,* and *NyQuil* are the most extensively advertised of this group.) These shotgun preparations contain in varying amounts and combinations a vasoconstrictor decongestant (phenylephrine or phenylpropanolamine), an antihistamine (chlorpheniramine or methapyrilene), an analgesic (aspirin or acetaminophen), a stimulant (caffeine), as well as vitamin C (ascorbic acid) and other ingredients. The medical profession has consistently repudiated this shotgun approach to medication, but has made little headway against the tide of publicity generated by the pharmaceutical industry.

CU's medical consultants have repeatedly stated that there are few categories of disease for which the use of a fixed combination is warranted — and the common cold is certainly not one of these. Most fixed-component formulations force the patient to take unnecessary medications. For example, the inclusion of antihistamines in a cold preparation is irrational, in the opinion of CU's medical consultants. As noted earlier, antihistamines have not been shown to be of value in the treatment of the common cold. Their inclusion in cold capsules "just on the chance that an allergy might be present" cannot be justified, especially in view of the major side effect — drowsiness — associated with their use. Antihistamines in cold capsules undoubtedly contribute to automobile accidents.

Aspirin (or some other analgesic or antipyretic) is often useful for a cold, but is not invariably required for all cold sufferers. Even though aches and pains do accompany a common cold — and a fever also does on rare occasions — aspirin must be taken in sufficient dosage to be effective. Some cold remedy formulations do not include amounts large enough to act effectively either as an analgesic or an antipyretic.

Of all the ingredients in a typical cold tablet, perhaps the most controversial is the oral decongestant. Some authorities believe that certain oral decongestants — in proper dosage — may help to relieve cold symptoms. On the other hand, the typical decongestants in most cold remedies do not work — either because they simply are ineffective or because the dose is too small to do any good.

Phenylephrine, for example, is the most widely used decongestant in nonprescription cold preparations. In clinical studies it has proved ineffective in oral doses up to 40 milligrams. Most OTC cold tablets or capsules containing phenylephrine have less than *half* that amount.

Among the fixed-combination products, the heaviest sales pitch goes for *Dristan Decongestant Tablets*, which rode a $12 million wave of advertising in 1972. "The exclusive *Dristan* formula cannot be duplicated," claims the package insert. According to its manufacturer, American Home Products, *Dristan* contains "the decongestant most prescribed by doctors," an "exclusive anti-allergent," and the "pain-relieving medication most recommended by doctors."

What is this remarkable formula? The decongestant is phenylephrine. And doctors do prescribe it often – but as *nose drops*, not orally. Moreover, the oral dose in two *Dristan* tablets (the recommended adult dosage) is only one-fourth of the amount found to be *ineffective* in controlled clinical testing. The "exclusive anti-allergent" is a relatively weak antihistamine, phenindamine. Its dosage in two *Dristan* tablets is less than that ordinarily given to children for hay fever. And like any antihistamine, it would be useless for cold symptoms.

The pain-reliever "most recommended by doctors" is, of course, aspirin. Each *Dristan* tablet contains the same amount as any 5-grain aspirin tablet. It is therefore true that *Dristan* does "work on aches and fever," as its television ads claim – but so does any aspirin. *Dristan* also includes a small amount of antacid and about as much caffeine per tablet as one ounce of brewed coffee. Neither of those ingredients relieves cold symptoms, however. In short, *Dristan* has only one effective aid for a cold: aspirin. But $12 million worth of advertising helped American Home Products sell *Dristan* for roughly twenty times the price of plain aspirin.

Alka-Seltzer Plus Cold Tablets contain much the same type of ingredients as *Dristan*: phenylephrine, antacids, an antihistamine (chlorpheniramine) and – aspirin. It has more antacid than *Dristan*, and it fizzes in a glass of water. But its sole value for cold symptoms is, again, 5 grains of aspirin. Like *Dristan*, *Alka-Seltzer Plus* sells for much more than unadorned aspirin.

Coricidin D, another shotgun cold tablet, rides much the same bandwagon. Again, there is phenylephrine, an antihistamine (chlorpheniramine), caffeine — and 6 grains of aspirin (instead of the usual 5). Curiously, the recommended dosage on the label is one tablet rather than two. Consequently, an adult taking *Coricidin D* as directed does not even get an effective dose of aspirin. So for that privilege of being instructed to take too little aspirin, the cold sufferer pays as much as thirty times the price of plain aspirin. *Coricidin* differs from *Coricidin D* in that it omits the ineffective decongestant. It comes in an impressive red tablet, however, which may ease the pain of paying about twenty times the price of aspirin.

Since 1971 a new group of products has emerged on television to minister to the sinuses. Such offerings as *Sinarest* and *Sine-Off* have now joined the older *Sinutab* in the television commercial war against sinus headache and congestion. Their ingredients reveal these medications to be cold preparations in disguise. Each of the three products contains a pain reliever, a decongestant, and an antihistamine. Since sinus headache and congestion are frequent symptoms of a cold, it is not surprising that the same standard remedies are offered. These types of sinus products ring up some $35 million in annual sales.

The greatest merchandising success of all the shotgun cold remedies, *Contac*, came up with a new twist to the formula — the timed-release capsule. But judging by its formula, the more people give their cash to *Contac*, the likelier they are to keep their colds themselves. In addition to chlorpheniramine, *Contac* contains small amounts of belladonna alkaloids. *Contac* also contains 50 milligrams of phenylpropanolamine, a decongestant that can indeed be helpful for a few hours at doses of 25 to 50 milligrams. Unfortunately, with *Contac's* timed-release formula, the dosage is theoretically spread out over twelve hours, so the user gets too meager a dose at any one time to be effective against cold symptoms.

35

Timed-release preparations have been used with dubious success for a variety of prescription drugs as well as OTC cold remedies. In a discussion of such dosage forms a few years ago, *The Medical Letter* commented, "Even with the most carefully formulated products, the rate of release in a particular patient is unpredictable. Release may be excessively rapid, or it can take an excessively lengthy period to obtain a sufficient dose of the drug. The widest variation in action must be expected with such medications." The Revision Committee of the U.S. Pharmacopeia (USP) has not recommended timed-release preparations for USP recognition, because it believes that no such form of any drug has been shown to be essential or valuable in medical practice. CU's medical consultants concur and advise against the use of timed-release preparations.

CU's medical consultants warn that those who take a shotgun remedy expose themselves to the allergic potential of not just one drug, but of several drugs. The miseries of the cold sufferer could then be compounded by a possible allergic reaction. And when the drugs are formulated into a timed-release preparation, the allergic reaction and accompanying discomfort can be prolonged. Similarly, side effects, which might ordinarily be short-lived, would also be prolonged.

One side effect of oral decongestants, which many people find intolerable, is excessive dryness in the nose, mouth, and throat. This uncomfortable sensation has caused many victims of colds to shy away from these products and to learn to tolerate their symptoms instead.

A warning is in order for certain cold sufferers who would be well advised to consult their physicians before using any decongestant preparation, either orally or as nose drops. Patients with hypertension (high blood pressure) should be aware that chemicals such as phenylpropanolamine and phenylephrine are "pressor" agents and are thus capable, in sufficient dosage, of causing elevation of blood pressure. Decongestants may also cause side effects in patients with thyroid disease and may alter the effect of insulin therapy in diabetics.

In 1970 interest in vitamin C was revived by Dr. Linus Pauling with the publication of his book, *Vitamin C and the Common Cold*. Dr. Pauling cited several experimental studies, anecdotal evidence, and personal experience to support his belief that large doses of vitamin C can prevent or cure the common cold and possibly other respiratory infections as well.

After careful scrutiny and thoughtful consideration, *The Medical Letter* and CU's medical consultants and statisticians judged that the studies cited were inadequately controlled. Differences in individual resistance and the natural course of an untreated respiratory infection, *The Medical Letter* noted, have an important bearing on the apparent effects of any proposed remedy. Thus a well-designed, controlled trial that is double-blind must be conducted over a sufficiently long period and must include hundreds of persons to give meaningful results.

One well-controlled study purporting to show the efficacy of vitamin C was published in Canada in September 1972. More than 800 people were involved in the double-blind study which extended over several months. Although the vitamin C group experienced slightly fewer colds and total days of illness, the difference was not statistically significant. The study did show, however, a significant reduction in the total number of days members of the vitamin C group lost from their jobs, because their illness was characterized by a "lower incidence of constitutional symptoms such as chills and severe malaise." A subsequent study by the Canadian researchers obtained similar results. (See "Is Vitamin C Really Good for Colds?" CONSUMER REPORTS, February 1976.)

A 1973 editorial in the *British Medical Journal* said about vitamin C that ". . . too little is known about the possible harmful effects of taking too much." While vitamin C has been promoted as "essentially nontoxic" and "harmless," CU's medical consultants are not so sure, particularly in view of the extremely large doses recommended in Dr. Pauling's book (over 300 times the recommended daily allowances now set by the Food and Nutrition Board of the National Research Council). Diarrhea to the point of being disabling can result from excessive doses of vitamin C. Some people, the pregnant (see below) and the elderly, for example, and those with certain illnesses — diagnosed or undiagnosed — might run even greater risks than the medically "normal" person.

Chronic urinary acidification, as is possible with the ingestion of 4 grams or more of vitamin C daily for months, may increase the frequency of kidney stones in persons disposed to gout. And ingestion of as much as 10 grams of vitamin C a day for several days might, in the judgment of some authorities, impose a formidable acid load on the body, especially on those with impaired kidney function. Also, the presence of large amounts of ascorbic acid in the urine interferes with urine sugar testing. Two popular methods currently employed by diabetics involve color reactions following the testing of urine with a tablet or paper tape. With the tablet (*Clinitest*) method, ascorbic acid can alter the color reaction and give an erroneous impression of excessive sugar in the urine. Diabetics who use *Testape* (a paper dip method) and take high doses of vitamin C may be falsely reassured because ascorbic acid interferes with the color reaction indicating sugar in the urine. Either of these incorrect results could thus cause some diabetics to change their medication dosage, with possibly serious consequences.

In addition, some authorities suspect that excessive vitamin C during pregnancy may result in infants who, despite normal intake of vitamin C after birth, may develop scurvy because their enzyme system had adjusted to high levels during the fetal period. Finally, the fad for vitamin C has led some persons to use a version of it containing sodium ascorbate, which could carry a special hazard for those on a low-sodium diet.

There is some evidence, on the basis of experiments with animals, to suggest that large doses of ascorbic acid may have detrimental effects on growing bone. At the present time there are no controlled studies that confirm this possibility in human beings who have been exposed to large doses of ascorbic acid over long periods of time.

Determining the extent of possible dangers — real and theoretical — accompanying a sustained large intake of vitamin C (250 to 15,000 milligrams daily over several months) calls for more extensive and better-controlled toxicity studies than are now available. Whatever the purported merits of increasing vitamin C allowances (and CU feels they should continue to be explored), toxicity studies should precede any efforts to encourage people to take large amounts of any substance, however seemingly innocuous.

Antibiotics, while not useful against colds themselves, are sometimes prescribed by physicians to prevent middle ear infection, sinusitis, bronchitis, or other complications of a common cold. Such dosing may not prevent these complications and might cause complications of its own, including an increase in bacterial resistance or an allergic reaction to the antibiotic itself. Of course, if a bacterial complication does occur — such as otitis (ear infection) or sinusitis — the timely use of an appropriate antibiotic may be helpful. (See Chapter 28 for a discussion of antibiotics.)

Still in the experimental stage is a material called interferon, a potential cold preventive, which is produced by body cells in response to many viral infections. So far, the substance is produced in such small amounts that large quantities of blood have to be processed in order to obtain sufficient interferon to treat a single individual. Methods for increasing body production of interferon, and procedures by which it can be synthesized, are currently being sought by researchers.

One authoritative appraisal of cold remedies was still not available as of this writing. A panel of scientists assembled by the FDA has evaluated more than 150 such products for safety and efficacy; its report was due in September 1976. The panel's findings may lead to FDA regulations on what should and should not be included in cold preparations.

Meanwhile, the question of what to do for a cold remains open. Resting in bed for a day or so, especially if symptoms are severe, may be a good idea — partly because rest may avert complications — but there is no real proof of the efficacy of bed rest in treating the common cold. Taking oneself out of circulation for a day or two may help prevent spreading the virus around. Recent evidence has incriminated the hands of a cold victim as an important factor in transmission of the virus. To minimize transmission of the cold virus, CU's medical consultants suggest that cold sufferers wash their hands frequently and avoid touching their eyes and nose for the duration of the cold. Although a handkerchief used for nose blowing is a relatively poor vehicle for spreading the virus, it makes sense to stick to throwaway paper tissues which cut down on the number of times the cold sufferer handles infected materials.

Some authorities endorse familiar folk remedies — chicken soup and aspirin — as being as effective as anything else. Decongestant nose drops (or nonaerosol nasal sprays) may provide transient relief for a stuffy nose and might also forestall ear complications by preventing blockage of the Eustachian tubes.

Research has demonstrated that decongestants are more effective when applied topically (as in nose drops) than when taken orally. CU's medical consultants suggest the judicious use of phenylephrine hydrochloride solution USP ½ percent (*Alcon-Efrin*, *Neo-Synephrine*, and various other brands); ¼ percent solution is recommended for infants and children. Since nose drops or spray may, after providing initial relief, actually worsen nasal congestion (rebound effect), use of such a product should be restricted to two or three times a day.

For those who can safely use a decongestant (see page 36), and prefer taking an oral one instead of nose drops or spray, the choice among OTC products may be limited. CU's medical consultants know of only two oral decongestants sold in effective dosages without a prescription. One is phenylpropanolamine (*Propadrine*), which has a decongestant effect at 25 to 50 milligrams. The other is pseudoephedrine (*Sudafed*), which is effective in dosages of 30 to 60 milligrams. These medications should be taken only as directed on the label. Phenylpropanolamine can also be purchased in a few combination products that include a pain reliever but no antihistamine. *Endecon, Ornex, Sine-Aid*, and *Sinutab-II* each offer that combination; some drugstores carry less expensive "house" brands with similar formulas.

Medical advice is rarely required for the common cold. What CU's medical consultants do recommend is patience, since most colds last from one to two weeks whether they are treated or not. In fact, some authorities believe that any attempt to suppress the symptoms of a cold may actually prolong the infection.

Chapter 3

Coughs
and
cough remedies

MORE THAN 800 OVER-THE-COUNTER (OTC) cough remedies are to be found on druggists' shelves, and about 100 additional cough mixtures compete for the doctor's prescription pad. With sales of these products so high, it is remarkable that reliable evidence of the effectiveness of popular cough remedies is virtually impossible to find. Indeed, some studies have indicated that, at least in chronic illness, even the more potent cough-depressant ingredients used in cough mixtures have no detectable effect at all on the cough itself, although patients treated with these drugs — or with a placebo — *think* they have improved. According to the editors of the *Journal of the American Medical Association*, "Neither practicing physicians nor [the] pharmaceutical industry can produce the objective evidence required under the law on behalf of most cough mixtures."

In fact, the Food and Drug Administration (FDA) served notice in February 1973 that it would ban more than twenty-five brands of fixed-combination cough medicines because of lack of evidence of their efficacy. An FDA review panel, charged with establishing the proper formulation and labeling of OTC preparations for coughs, colds, and allergies, has not reported its findings as of this writing (see page 40). Its recommendations may well have a tremendous impact on the $735 million market for cough and cold remedies.

Coughing is a multiple-stage reflex action controlled by a cough center in the brain which responds to irritation in the respiratory tract. Coughing performs an important protective function by both loosening and expectorating secretions, and may even be lifesaving when used to expel a foreign object. Coughing may also be a nervous act, as in clearing one's throat prior to delivering a speech. A cough can become a disabling ticlike disorder, which may respond to a tranquilizing drug. In other words, coughing is a symptom which may have any one of a number of causes — some innocuous, others serious.

The most frequent and, fortunately, one of the most innocent causes of coughing is the common cold. Most effects of a cold ordinarily go away in a week or two, with or without treatment (see Chapter 2). But a cough accompanying a common cold can be a nuisance. Coughing can usually be relieved by sucking plain hard candies, by drinking hot beverages, or by inhaling steam. Any of these should help limit the frequency and severity of coughing. A cough lingering longer than a week following a cold merits a visit to a physician.

Although tobacco smoke affects people in different ways, heavy smoking unquestionably causes many a cough. Even in a chain smoker, however, it should never be assumed without a thorough medical examination that a cough is caused simply by smoking. The most pernicious aspect of the advertising of cough remedies is that many "smoker's coughs" and "coughs following a cold" may be associated with more serious diseases of the respiratory tract. Such diseases as pneumonia, bronchitis, cancer, or heart failure may be real but unsuspected causes of acute or persistent coughing.

When a cough is caused by an infection, there are remedies that can help; in the case of a cough due to pneumonia, for instance, specific antibiotics can effectively treat the underlying disease and thereby relieve the cough. It is unusual, however, for a cough to be given such rational treatment. One way or another, a cough remedy generally gets into the act, usually at the outset and often before the underlying cause of the cough is diagnosed. Although many cough mixtures depress the appetite or even cause nausea, they usually do no harm (in recommended doses), they taste pleasant, and they often have a soothing psychological effect. Coughing patients are prone to demand *something* from their doctors, and doctors are often loath to deny a patient the psychological comfort a remedy may provide.

Advertising claims by makers of cough and cold remedies led to demands by the Federal Trade Commission (FTC) for substantiation. In January 1973 the FTC released documents submitted by sixteen manufacturers of thirty-five cough and cold remedies. The public learned, among other things, that *Father John's Medicine* was not — despite wording in ads — prepared according to a doctor's prescription after all, that *Pertussin Plus Night-Time Cold Medicine* "must be used with caution during the day" because of its antihistamine content (which can induce drowsiness), and that *St. Joseph Cough Syrup for Children* — despite its name — does not claim its product is made especially for children.

Most cough mixtures, whether OTC or prescription, are shotgun remedies (see page 32), containing from two to perhaps ten different drugs aimed at the various links in the cough mechanism. The ingredients can, it is alleged, combat allergies, decrease (or increase) the secretion of mucus, stimulate the sympathetic nervous system, inhibit the parasympathetic nervous system, tranquilize (or stimulate) the patient, depress the cough center in the brain, or depress peripheral nerve reflexes. The theory seems to be that, if you use enough ingredients, at least one should work.

The ingredients with the most significant effects in typical OTC cough mixtures are sugar and alcohol — the former acting as a demulcent, which seems to relieve sore, irritated mucous membranes, and the latter acting as a mild depressant of the central nervous system. (Sugar-free medications are also available for diabetics.) Alcohol constitutes 25 percent of *Creo-Terpin*, *NyQuil*, and *Pertussin Plus Night-Time Cold Medicine*; 20 percent of *Cosadein*; 15 percent of *Coldene Cough Formula Adult* and *Trind*; and 12 percent of *Dristan Cough Formula*.

The label for *NyQuil* suggests taking the medicine at bedtime, because it "relieves major cold symptoms for hours to let you get the restful sleep your body needs." Two of the ingredients in *NyQuil* may help to induce sleep — but not by relieving cold symptoms. The alcohol content of *NyQuil* makes the drink 50 proof, and the antihistamine in it (doxylamine succinate) is known as a cause of drowsiness. Unfortunately, *NyQuil* has too little medication to relieve congestion, which is often what hinders sleep for the cold victim. Its 8 milligrams of ephedrine are less than one-third of the dose usually prescribed for effective decongestant action. Ephedrine is also a central nervous system stimulant, which can work against the product's sedative effect even at the low dosage level. *NyQuil* does contain a cough suppressant that might help someone sleep. But that action may be counteracted by the antihistamine, which can intensify a cough by thickening bronchial secretions. In short, *NyQuil* seems to be just the thing for cold sufferers in search of a medication that might knock them out, wake them up, and suppress their cough while worsening it.

In addition to sugar and alcohol, other frequently used ingredients in cough mixtures are codeine (a narcotic, not used for OTC cough products in some states), dextromethorphan (a nonnarcotic similar in action to codeine), ammonium and iodide salts, glycerol, and flavorings of all kinds. Codeine and dextromethorphan, in the amounts present in cough remedies, probably do exert a mild depressant action on the cough center in the brain, but they can also cause nausea and drowsiness in a significant number of users. And if cough suppressants are taken in doses sufficiently large to suppress the cough reflex, they may also discourage the expectoration or loosening of secretions. This, of course, can be harmful.

In May 1973 the FDA published proposed guidelines for the reformulation and relabeling of prescription cough preparations. The FDA cited as its "regulatory philosophy" the belief that medications should include only ingredients of proven effectiveness for the symptomatic relief of common ailments. Accordingly, the FDA stated that it would no longer permit three categories of ingredients in cough preparations. The 1973 guidelines would ban analgesics, such as aspirin or acetaminophen, from these medications, and would no longer permit antihistamines and oral decongestants in prescription cough remedies. Not unexpectedly, the Pharmaceutical Manufacturers Association has attacked these proposed guidelines for prescription remedies.

The amounts of the various expectorants in popular cough remedies — ammonium chloride, ammonium carbonate, potassium iodide, ipecac, guaiacolate, and terpin hydrate, among others — are so small that they are hardly capable of influencing a cough. In fact, the FDA in its May 1973 interim guidelines no longer permits some kinds of expectorants in prescription cough preparations because they lack effectiveness and/or are unsafe. When the findings of the panel on OTC cough and cold preparations are made available, the FDA warns that it may then add to its list of prohibited expectorants, should the panel judge other expectorants "to be less than effective."

The psychological value of most cough remedies, however, must be emphasized. Dr. Henry K. Beecher, of the Harvard Medical School, showed that many patients with coughs due to diseases of the respiratory tract derive great psychological satisfaction from cough remedies, even when it has been objectively demonstrated that the remedies failed to reduce either the frequency or the intensity of the cough.

In other words, when cough remedies work, they usually do so by altering the patient's emotional state in such a way as to reduce the anxiety about the cough and to induce a belief that objective improvement has resulted. If a person with a cough believes in the remedy, that person probably can obtain as much relief from a simple, inexpensive product as from the most elaborate and costly one.

A vaporizer can help relieve the dry cough that sometimes accompanies a cold. Its sole job is to put a lot of moisture into the air to loosen secretions in the upper respiratory tract. In 1973 CU tested three types of electric vaporizers: the cool-mist, the electrolytic, and the boiler. All seventeen models of the cool-mist type were found Acceptable; three of the eight electrolytic models were rated Acceptable. One example of a boiler vaporizer tested was found to be relatively safe, but slow. There is no difference, therapeutically, in the effect of warm moisture over cool. However, the electrolytic (or steam) type of vaporizer offers some advantages — including more initial relief-giving moisture — but is not as safe to use as the cool-mist models because of the potential for severe shock. The hazard in using the cool-mist type of vaporizer is in the maintenance of the unit. Special care must be taken to use fresh water each time and to wash the reservoir thoroughly before each refilling to prevent the growth of bacteria and fungi within the reservoir. The boiler vaporizer offers the possibility of steam without the shock potential of the electrolytic, although it takes much longer than the other two types of vaporizers to get going.

Adding an aromatic product such as *Vicks VapoSteam* or *Vicks VapoRub* to a steam vaporizer provides no additional benefit and may possibly introduce a hazard. In a study presented to the American College of Chest Physicians in October 1973, laboratory animals exposed to steam vapors of *Vicks VapoRub* were reported to experience a decline in their natural defenses against bacterial infection. It is not known whether such an effect would also apply to human beings. But CU's medical consultants point out that there is no sense in taking chances with a product that has no proven value anyway.

Some authorities favor the use of old-fashioned remedies — mixtures of whiskey, honey, and lemon juice, or of hot milk and honey. Medicated lozenges and so-called cough drops are very popular items in the OTC cough-remedy market. In 1973 about 43 billion cough drops reportedly were sold in this country. These products contain varying combinations of glycerine, honey, cocilana, camphor, menthol, eucalyptus oil, and flavoring agents. CU's medical consultants believe that such cough drops offer no advantages over less expensive hard candies.

For a cough that lasts longer than a week, a doctor's help should be sought. For chronic coughs, cough remedies and self-medication are not a good idea. There is evidence that the long-continued use of a cough medicine containing a narcotic or one containing a high percentage of alcohol leads to what Dr. Beecher euphemistically calls "an unusual degree of satisfaction in their use." Most doctors, therefore, discourage prolonged use of such remedies for chronic coughs. Some patients in whom thorough medical investigation has failed to reveal a treatable cause of their coughing are able to adapt themselves to a chronic cough, even though they have to cough many times a day.

Chapter 4

Sore throats

A SORE THROAT can be quite disabling. Each swallow of saliva, food, or drink can serve as a cruel reminder. The common postnasal drip, which may be the result of a chronic sinus infection or an allergy, can cause severe throat irritation. In winter some sore throats can be traced to insufficient humidity due to overheated houses and closed windows. Breathing through the mouth while sleeping can also cause excessive dryness of the mucous membranes. These kinds of sore throats can be avoided by humidification or by eliminating the cause of mouth breathing (by consultation with a physician, if necessary). Dryness of the mucous membranes may predispose one to infections of the upper respiratory tract. In fact, some ear, nose, and throat specialists believe that proper humidification can actually decrease the incidence of throat infections.

The most common cause of a sore throat is infection, and more of these throat infections are viral than bacterial in origin. However, it is often difficult to tell them apart; a fever, for instance, may characterize both types. Any doubts can usually be resolved by means of blood counts and throat cultures, if necessary. The familiar "strep throat" (caused by streptococci bacteria) may sometimes be distinguished by yellowish pus which covers the tonsils. Unfortunately for diagnostic purposes, this appearance can be mimicked by certain viruses, such as the virus that causes infectious mononucleosis.

It is not merely a matter of academic interest to distinguish between bacterial and viral sore throats. If untreated, a strep throat can lead to heart or kidney damage. A ten-day course of penicillin is the treatment of choice for strep throat. (If there is a history of allergy to the drug, other antibiotics are used — see Chapter 28.) Occasionally, other bacteria such as staphylococci or gonococci may cause sore throats, but streptococci account for most bacterial infections.

Viral sore throats are less easy to identify, because culture techniques for detecting viruses are much more complicated and are usually not practicable. Some viruses, such as herpes or Coxsackie, often cause small painful ulcerations, commonly called canker sores, on the tongue and in the mouth.

A healthy mouth and throat contain myriads of bacteria and other organisms. The collective name given this germ population is "normal flora." Usually, none of these organisms causes disease. Occasionally, a healthy person may be a carrier of disease-producing bacteria, such as streptococci or staphylococci. When the organism — not readily identifiable in its host's mouth or throat — comes in contact with a susceptible individual, it transfers to the more inviting situation and an infection is initiated by this invasion of the tissues of the throat. The precise reason why one person is resistant and another vulnerable is poorly understood.

Once bacteria or viruses initiate an infection, the tissues of the throat react to combat it. Blood vessels dilate to increase blood flow to the area, bringing blood cells that act as scavengers. The increased blood flow causes the mucous membranes to redden and the underlying tissues to swell. It is the swelling that is primarily responsible for pain. In a severe sore throat there may be spasms of the throat muscles, which serve to increase discomfort.

Use of an antiseptic gargle or medicated lozenges can do little to cure the infection. The offending organisms are deep in the throat tissues, and it is only by means of an appropriate antibiotic in sufficient dosage (taken by mouth or by injection) that adequate amounts of medication can be delivered to the infected area via the bloodstream.

Even less rational is the use of medicated gargles, mouthwashes, or lozenges as sore throat *preventives.* Any antiseptic action of these products is momentary at best, because of the impossibility of sterilizing the oral cavity. The full complement of "normal flora" can be easily restored with the next few breaths, a quick kiss, or even a lick of the lips.

In 1970 the Food and Drug Administration (FDA) served notice that it would no longer permit manufacturers of mouthwashes to claim that their products were of any medicinal value. The agency ordered the manufacturers of eight mouthwashes to cease claiming that mouthwashes could stop bad breath (see Chapter 15), kill germs, or combat colds. The action followed a report prepared for the FDA by the National Academy of Sciences–National Research Council. The mouthwash study found no convincing evidence that mouthwashes have any medicinal advantage over water.

The mouthwashes affected by the FDA announcement were *Betadine Mouthwash/Gargle, Cepacol Mouthwash Gargle, Isodine Gargle and Mouthwash, Kasdenol Mouthwash and Gargle, Micrin Oral Antiseptic, Pepsodent Antiseptic Mouthwash, Sterisol Mouthwash,* and *Tyrolaris Mouthwash.* Pending a final report on over-the-counter (OTC) preparations, mouthwashes were permitted in 1971 to claim "to help provide soothing temporary relief of dryness and minor irritations of the mouth and throat."

One of the biggest-selling mouthwashes, *Listerine Antiseptic,* was not directly affected by the FDA order because it was put on the market before 1938. Congress had strengthened the

Food, Drug, and Cosmetic Act in 1962 by requiring manufacturers to prove their claims for the effectiveness of new drugs
and all drugs introduced since 1938. But no further clearance
was required for older drugs. The FDA, therefore, has turned
to the Federal Trade Commission to monitor advertising claims
for *Listerine* and several other pre-1938 mouthwashes on the
ground that the mouthwash study's findings are equally applicable to them.

How about the action of gargles against the *pain* of a sore
throat? Here the case is not as clear. It is possible that some
gargles might provide relief of inflammatory pain as a result
of an astringent effect on surface congestion or of a transient
anesthetic effect, although CU's medical consultants know of
no controlled studies that have tested these possibilities. In fact,
the mechanical act of gargling may bring some benefit to the
inflamed throat, independent of the specific composition of the
gargling solution.

CU's medical consultants recommend warm salt water (one-
half teaspoon of table salt to an 8-ounce glass of warm water)
both as a gargle and a mouthwash. This mildly concentrated
salt solution may help to reduce the painful swelling. In addition, aspirin taken by mouth (but not as a gargle — see page
15) may be helpful in relieving general discomfort. Occasionally, for the pain of a very sore throat a physician may prescribe
a mild narcotic such as codeine tablets.

Insistent advertising has pressured many people suffering
from a sore throat to swallow some improbable ideas about
the efficacy of the gargles, mouthwashes, rinsing solutions,
lozenges, and even medicated chewing gum filling pharmacy
and supermarket shelves. One example is the case put forward
for *Aspergum*. This chewing gum product is touted as being
capable of bringing "fast temporary relief of minor sore throat
pain." In fact, topical treatment of sore throats is one of the
few tasks aspirin cannot tackle in terms of pain-relief capacity.

The failure of OTC sore throat remedies to live up to the implications of their well-hedged claims is one thing; a more serious basis for criticism is the occasional real harm they may foster. When people are induced to dose a sore throat with a patent medicine, they may be delaying proper diagnosis and treatment by a physician.

As noted earlier, untreated throat infections caused by streptococci can cause heart or kidney damage. Even though many, perhaps most, sore throats are caused by viruses — and not by bacteria — the user of a patent medicine has no way of telling what brought on a particular sore throat. If the sore throat should prove to be viral in origin, the consequences are usually not serious. But the gamble involved in not checking into the cause of the sore throat can be risky, should the infection be bacterial and diagnosis delayed by dependence on OTC medications.

Lozenges are also extensively promoted for relief of pain from sore throats. These preparations usually contain a topical anesthetic such as benzocaine. At best, the pain relief obtained from use of a lozenge is short-lived. And what is more, any transitory benefits may be offset by the possibility of an allergic reaction to the ingredients in the lozenge.

CU's medical consultants summarize as follows their recommendations for treating a sore throat:

- Avoid all OTC remedies.
- Gargle with warm salt water.
- Take ordinary aspirin for general discomfort.
- If the sore throat lasts more than a day or two or is accompanied by fever, check with a doctor.

Chapter 5

Care of the teeth and gums

LOSS OT TEETH need not go hand in hand with aging. But the statistics are not encouraging. Authorities estimate that more than 50 percent of all Americans are toothless by the age of sixty-five. Much of that loss is unnecessary. With the use of available preventive techniques and proper dental care, started soon enough, most people can chew with their own teeth for as long as they live.

Tooth decay and pyorrhea, the most common dental ills leading to loss of teeth, are complex diseases having many aspects which are as yet poorly understood. While both are essentially bacterial diseases, they result typically from an interplay of forces — not necessarily from a specific germ, dietary deficiency, or other single cause. Researchers have not yet precisely determined the importance of each element that contributes to the onset, severity, and ultimate outcome of these diseases. The broad outlines, however, are fairly well known.

TOOTH DECAY

Tooth decay (dental caries) is a disease that afflicts at least 95 percent of Americans. The interaction of three factors is chiefly responsible for caries: bacterial plaque, certain carbohydrates (primarily processed sugar), and an hospitable tooth surface.

Plaque is formed in several stages. The first occurs when a "film" (or pellicle), derived mainly from saliva, develops on the tooth surface. The pellicle becomes full-fledged plaque when it is colonized by streptococci and other bacteria which go to work on sugars and other food particles retained in the mouth. One of the resulting by-products of bacterial activity on sugar is dextran, a thick gel-like material, which sticks tenaciously to the surface of the teeth and hastens plaque buildup unless removed by careful prophylactic measures (see page 68). Sugar-rich food residue in the mouth not only is the source of dextran; more importantly, it can also be broken down rapidly by bacteria to form acid. Plaque holds the acid against the tooth surface. There the acid attacks the tooth with a success that depends on the tooth's vulnerability to decay. The acid forms to a much greater extent in the mouths of individuals who are highly susceptible to dental decay. The factors responsible for increased resistance to dental decay are largely unknown; one possibility is that they are genetic in origin. Theoretically, anything that prevents production of acid, neutralizes it, removes it quickly from the mouth, or helps the tooth to resist its action should reduce decay.

One approach to prevention of acid formation is a direct attack on the mouth's streptococcal bacteria. However, some authorities believe that only a small percentage of the total streptococcal bacteria present in the mouth actually account for dental decay. Unfortunately, the mouth harbors such enormous numbers of bacteria, and they are so well sheltered by successive overlays of plaque, that it is difficult to immobilize enough bacteria — safely — to reduce acid formation significantly.

Limited success with the antibacterial approach has been demonstrated through daily use of an antiseptic mouthwash, chlorhexidine gluconate, which binds to the surface of the teeth. Research with Scandinavian volunteers demonstrated that it is possible to achieve almost total prevention of plaque, calculus (see below), and of gingival — or gum — disease (see page 64) for as long as 150 days. Additional research with a dentifrice containing chlorhexidine suggests that some reduction in dental caries can also be expected. However, experiments with animals showed that after six months plaque began to return, despite continued use of the solution. Concerns have also arisen about side effects from long-term use. In the United States the Food and Drug Administration (FDA) has authorized the use of chlorhexidine for clinical tests, but as of this writing no applications have been filed with the FDA for products containing the drug.

How about going after the soft, sticky plaque that holds the acid to the teeth? Easier said than done. Plaque differs greatly from person to person — sometimes neutralizing the acid, and sometimes helping it to form. Plaque accumulates constantly, and it seems to do so faster in decay-prone people than in those resistant to caries. Researchers now agree that plaque is also the forerunner of calculus (popularly known as tartar), a hard substance which contributes to pyorrhea, a disease of the gums (see page 63).

Another avenue of attack on the decay problem involves dextran, the sticky material that helps the bacteria adhere to each other and to the tooth surface. In recent animal studies an enzyme, dextranase, has been found to break down dextran and reduce the ability of streptococci to generate plaque and cause tooth decay. However, dextranase by itself has been found to be minimally effective for human use, although it could conceivably become part of a systematic approach to fighting decay. But the findings are still in the experimental stage; there is no firm evidence that they apply to human beings.

The best day-to-day defense against plaque — and food debris as well — is careful attention to oral cleanliness. And you can help by cutting down your intake of sweets. Decay-causing bacteria thrive on candy, soft drinks, cookies, presweetened cereals, and other processed-sugar foods. Acid builds up very fast in the mouth after you eat sweets. People whose teeth decay readily would be wise to stick to fruit, and such snacks as celery or carrot sticks, for between-meal eating to help reduce exposure to rapid acid formation.

As of now, toughening the teeth themselves against decay seems by far the most promising way to reduce the incidence of caries. Years of research have uncovered just one substance that authorities generally agree can do the job with high effectiveness — fluoride.

Fluoride can help build a decay-resistant tooth surface when painted onto teeth (so-called topical application). In addition, prophylactic dental paste with fluoride — material reserved by the FDA for the exclusive use of dentists or hygienists to clean teeth — has been shown to reduce tooth decay. Although theoretically there is no age limit in the use of topical applications of fluoride or of fluoride dentifrices, there is probably a falling-off of effectiveness with age. Studies so far have established only that fluoride works effectively when used by the young, including adolescents and young adults. CU's dental consultants believe that more study is needed to determine the degree of effectiveness in older people.

Fluoride does the best job, however, when it is included in proper amounts in the diet of growing children. As a practical matter, only one way to include it has proved to be highly effective, safe, and inexpensive for large-scale use — fluoridation of a community's water system. Children who drink fluoridated water for the first twelve years of their lives average 60 percent less decay than those who grow up without benefit of fluoride. The resistance to decay continues throughout life. There is also some evidence of enhanced resistance for those

57

who continued to drink fluoridated water into early adulthood.

Evidence, already voluminous, continues to pile up that fluoride in the relatively small amounts needed for decay prevention is safe for people of all ages and for the chronically ill — except for certain kidney patients (see page 59) — as well as for the healthy, and that fluoridation of a community's water supply is by far the best measure now available to bring about a drastic cut in the incidence of tooth decay. Some authorities believe that fluoride may be of limited use in the treatment of osteoporosis, a bone disease occurring frequently in older men and women. In fact, the Food and Nutrition Board of the National Research Council has now classified fluoride as "an essential nutrient."

The effectiveness of fluoride against tooth decay is seldom disputed anymore; by now the point is too well documented. Indeed, nine states already have legislation requiring municipalities to fluoridate their water supplies. The annual per-capita cost of community fluoridation is only a fraction of the cost of filling a tooth. Despite this fact, community water fluoridation still arouses bitter opposition in certain areas of the United States — some of it based on misunderstandings about the safety of flouride, and some on philosophical objections. Some opponents of fluoridation point to studies purporting to show that fluoride causes a host of ills ranging from mouth ulcers and migraine headaches to mongolism and cancer. According to CU's dental and medical consultants, there is no valid evidence for the purported harmful effects of low-level fluoridation.

It is true that fluoride is toxic. But it is toxic only in high concentrations which have no relevance to the amounts taken in by drinking from an optimally fluoridated water supply. Fluoride is often present in natural water, sometimes at relatively high levels. One study compared a community with a percentage of natural fluoride in the water of 0.4 parts per million with another community naturally fluoridated at 8 parts per million — eight times the 1-part-per-million recommendation of the U.S. Public Health Service (PHS). By the end of the study, the participants had been exposed to fluoridation for at least twenty-five years. Another study followed the children of two cities, one fluoridated and the other not, for a decade. In these and other studies, no fluoride-related bone abnormalities, pathological effects, or differences in death rate showed up.

Fluoridated water can cause whitish or brownish stains on the teeth of some children. But at the recommended 1-part-per-million level, only a small percentage of children is affected, and the mottling is so slight that it takes a trained eye to detect it. Questions have been raised about the safety of fluoridated tap water for patients with severe or total kidney impairment. Indeed, the National Institute of Arthritis and Metabolic Disease (a division of the PHS) recommends that fluoride — as well as calcium, magnesium, and copper — be removed from tap water *before it is used in an artificial kidney machine*. This recommendation is based on the fact that a kidney patient who needs such dialysis treatment two to three times a week is thereby exposed to about 50 to 100 times the amount of fluid consumed by the average person. It has no bearing, the PHS says, on the ingestion by *anyone* of optimally fluoridated water from a community water supply.

Nevertheless, CU believes that reports of adverse effects, however isolated and of whatever validity, should not be ignored by the scientific community. For those concerned with public health, there is an obvious responsibility to keep a continuous watch over the effects of such a widespread practice as fluoridation.

Those who oppose community fluoridation on principle, while admitting the value of dietary fluoride, sometimes suggest that individuals who want fluoride could add it to food at home. This would be neither as simple nor as reliable and safe as fluoridation of community water. Although the use of tablets containing fluoride, or its addition to the family drinking water or to fruit juice, has been shown to be an effective procedure, it is certainly more costly and complex for a family. For one thing, a prescription from a doctor or dentist would be required. Since the water in many communities already contains some natural fluoride, each family would have to measure out its own fluoride individually to adapt to the level of fluoride in the local water supply. There would be a problem in making sure that every child obtained enough, but not too much, of the fluoride-bearing food or drink.

The use of tablets containing fluoride obviously poses serious problems not found with community fluoridation. To obtain enough fluoride, children would have to drink all their water at home, or carry fluoridated water when they went out — a totally impractical regimen to follow. Excessive or prolonged doses of fluoride can be harmful, so parents would have to be careful in preparing the mixture and in storing the tablets out of the reach of children. Tablets taken directly would, of course, require supervision. And for maximum benefit, a family would have to go to all the fuss and bother for each child, every single day from birth until at least twelve years of age — and make sure that the tablets (or mixture) were taken faithfully.

Where water fluoridation is not available on a community-wide basis, another possibility is treatment of the water supply at a local public school by the addition of fluoride at a slightly higher level than usual, since the water is used only part time during school hours. Such procedures have brought a 35 to 40 percent reduction in caries, compared with the incidence in a control group. Fluoride mouthwashes, used in a controlled double-blind study, have also proven to be effective in reducing caries (by as much as 25 to 30 percent in some cases). Another alternative, one still in the experimental stage, is the possibility of adding fluoride to table salt. A World Health Organization study in 1972 reported that this technique may prove to be a safe, low-cost, and effective method of fluoridation.

Although fluoride functions most reliably when ingested, children can receive some benefits from fluoride even if they use water from private wells or live in communities that have not yet begun to fluoridate. Even when fluoridated water is used, many dentists recommend that youngsters receive topical applications of fluoride on their teeth until the eruption of the third molar (wisdom tooth). The disadvantage of such topical applications is that they ordinarily must be performed in a dental office or clinic by a dentist or dental hygienist. Such treatments are recommended on at least a yearly basis for those with average teeth; for those highly susceptible to tooth decay, more frequent treatments may be needed, perhaps continuing until the patients are in their twenties.

Three fluoride compounds commonly used by dentists are fluoride-phosphate, stannous fluoride, and sodium fluoride. Studies have indicated that fluoride-phosphate and stannous fluoride are about equal in efficacy; either may be somewhat more effective than sodium fluoride. Some dentists prefer fluoride-phosphate because the process of application is easier with it. Research is currently underway on a new generation of fluorides which, in combination with other chemicals, are designed to affect not only tooth surfaces but also the plaque associated with pyorrhea (see page 65).

Fluoride-phosphate can be applied in gel form via a specially made mouth guard which is worn about five minutes a day. When used under supervision for five days a week over a two-year period, this technique resulted in an average reduction of 85 percent fewer caries than in a control group. In an attempt to bypass the complicated and expensive requirement for individually designed guards, manufacturers have developed preformed models in standardized sizes, which depend on "spacers" to eliminate the slack and use a viscous gel which adheres closely to the teeth. Whether the procedure will prove as effective with these devices still remains to be determined, along with other questions, such as the optimal frequency for use of self-applied gels.

A less effective method of topical application is regular use of special fluoride toothpaste. The American Dental Association (ADA) recognizes four fluoride toothpastes as effective in reducing cavities: *Colgate MFP*, *Crest Mint*, *Crest Regular*, and, as of 1976, *Macleans Fluoride*. Those under twenty-five should normally make their choice of toothpaste from this group, since clinical studies have shown their effectiveness. For those who may be sensitive to some of the ingredients in these products, or to their taste, the following additional fluoride toothpastes were judged from CU's 1972 laboratory tests to have some decay-inhibiting potential: *A & P Fluoride*, *Gleem II*, *Rexall Fluoride*, *Safeway Fluoride*, and *Worthmore Stannous Fluoride*.

CU's dental consultants advise all adults to use fluoride toothpaste, but suggest that those with receding gums should first check with their dentists because such pastes might prove too abrasive. For a more extensive discussion of toothpastes, see page 68.

A fluoride toothpaste is helpful even when fluoride is also available from other sources. Some clinical studies suggest that regular use of a recommended fluoride dentifrice can prolong the effectiveness of a dentist's topical fluoride treatments. In fact, there are indications that both the use of a fluoride toothpaste and of topical applications are valuable even when fluoridated drinking water is available. CU's dental and medical consultants state that proper topical applications and fluoride toothbrushing do not increase the body's intake of fluoride beyond recommended limits, and do not present any danger of fluoride toxicity to those already drinking fluoridated water. Minute traces of additional fluoride, which might be swallowed with saliva, are not believed to pose any threat to health.

CU's dental and medical consultants recommend the multiple use of fluorides:

- Systemically (in water or as a dietary supplement);
- In topical application;
- In a dentifrice.

Those with rampant caries — and this is a small percentage — would be wise to check with their dentists about the supplemental use of a self-applied gel and a fluoride mouthwash, both available by prescription.

The latest approach to the prevention of tooth decay involves the use of a sealant, a plastic material that is painted onto the biting surfaces of the teeth. The physical barrier thus provided prevents plaque accumulation and the formation of caries. Tests with one variety of sealant showed that for about two years it can be highly effective, resulting in 80 to 90 percent less decay during that period. However, the usefulness of this procedure is largely confined to children, because their biting surfaces are highly susceptible to decay. CU's dental consultants believe sealants may have limited value, even for children, because of the possible need for repeated applications. And adults are certainly better off sticking with the standard prophylactic measures and, as soon as decay develops, having their teeth filled with a standard type of permanent filling.

PYORRHEA

Even if it were possible to make sure that children entered adult life with decay-free teeth, the battle for dental health would not be over. The other major enemy of teeth is perhaps even more insidious.

Dental decay most vigorously attacks children and young adults. If you're past thirty-five, the teeth you lose will most likely be lost to pyorrhea (periodontal disease). Like tooth decay, pyorrhea is a bacterial plaque disorder. However, it affects not the teeth themselves but the periodontium — the periodontal fibers, gums, and bone that support the teeth. Bleeding and swollen gums are the first warning signs you are likely to notice; irritation — mechanical (see page 65) as well as bacterial — is a frequent cause.

In its early stages, periodontal disease is called gingivitis, and it affects only the gums, or gingiva; if corrected at this time, the disease is reversible.

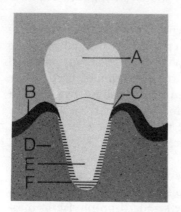 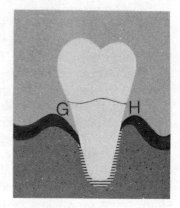

Effects of pyorrhea

Left: A tooth with normal support. Notice that only the crown (A) is exposed. The root (E) is completely enveloped in bone (D) to which it is held by a system of fibers called the periodontal membrane (F). Overlying the bone is the gingiva, or gum tissue (B), which hugs the tooth tightly, leaving only a shallow gingival crevice (C). The tooth at the right shows the effects of damage. The gingival crevice has deepened, and a periodontal pocket (G) has formed. The gingival recession (H) has also exposed parts of the root, and the reduced area of bone support permits the tooth to loosen.

Pyorrhea virtually always starts with plaque along the gum line. The plaque often becomes mineralized by calcium salts from saliva, thereby forming deposits of calculus. White in the initial stages, these deposits tend to change color to light yellow and then to dark brown, depending on eating and smoking habits and how long the deposits remain in the mouth. They first collect in protected areas around the necks of the teeth, most heavily inside the lower incisors and outside the upper molars — areas near the openings of the salivary gland ducts.

The plaque associated with gum disease is similar to the plaque involved in tooth decay, although often thicker and made up of a more complex mixture of bacteria. In the thick plaque associated with pyorrhea, a variety of bacteria produces several noxious products (e.g., toxins and some enzymes), which start a destructive chain reaction in the gums, and in time in the underlying supporting tissues of the teeth as well (see diagram).

When plaque hardens into calculus, an additional irritant is created — a mechanical irritant, affecting the gums every time you chew, swallow, or brush your teeth. Improperly made or overhanging fillings can have a similar effect. Impacted food residue, retained where the gum meets the tooth, often adds to the abrasive action and increases the irritation. Food also encourages still more bacteria to grow in the plaque, and blood from the gums provides excellent nutrients for the bacteria. The result: inflammation first, and then destruction of gum tissue.

As time passes, the gum tissue separates from the teeth, and a gingival crevice forms and deepens (see diagram). Plaque and calculus continue to form, extending the bacterial irritation down into the gingival crevice. The healthy, pink gum tissue that normally hugs the tooth and terminates in a fine margin takes on a swollen, bluish-red, blunted appearance and often becomes tender.

There are more serious consequences. The periodontal membrane, the system of fibers that connects the tooth's root to the supporting bone, becomes detached. The alveolar bone, the bone that forms the tooth socket, becomes infected, and is more and more seriously damaged. Plaque and calculus form ever deeper in the gingival pocket, extending the areas of local infection and inflammation. As increasing amounts of bone are lost from the socket, the tooth has less and less support. The tooth gradually loosens and, unless the process is halted, eventually falls out.

Bad alignment of the teeth may also contribute to pyorrhea. In a well-formed arch, the teeth are arranged evenly and symmetrically, those in the upper jaw meshing properly with the ones in the lower. Adjacent teeth that line up irregularly in the jaw, or teeth in the two opposing jaws that do not contact each other correctly, may set up any of several vicious cycles. They promote retention of dental plaque, since uneven teeth are often hard to clean and their grinding surfaces clean themselves less efficiently than those of properly meshing teeth. They also make it easier for stringy foods such as ham, chicken, or steak to become wedged between the teeth, where they may produce chronic gum irritation.

Furthermore, tilted, rotated, or otherwise malposed teeth subject the periodontal structures to abnormal stresses during chewing, which may contribute to a breakdown of the supporting bone. (For that matter, some fairly evenly distributed stresses can also be harmful. Nervous habits — such as frequent clenching of the teeth, lip or cheek biting, and compulsive tongue pressure against the teeth — can contribute to pyorrhea.)

Dental decay that advances far enough to affect tooth position can be a most important factor in pyorrhea. When a tooth is lost to decay, teeth next to the empty space tend to drift toward it. The opposing tooth in the other jaw is also inclined toward the vacant area. In its new position, a tooth that has drifted is inclined, rotated, or extended beyond the level of the other teeth. Spaces between nearby teeth widen, allowing food to collect there and irritate the gums.

If you lose several teeth and don't have them replaced, the remaining teeth may drift so extensively that they no longer function properly. Such a collapse of the entire occlusion produces enough undesirable leverage on the malposed teeth and strain on the supporting structures to affect adversely the supporting bone. The teeth become increasingly mobile, and the destructive forces continue to act on teeth whose ability to withstand them progressively decreases.

Cigarette smoking, too, is likely to promote gum disease. In 1968 a study of seven thousand people by Roswell Park Memorial Institute, Buffalo, New York, showed that the average periodontal condition of smokers was comparable to that of nonsmokers fifteen years their senior. Dental prospects for young women who smoke were found to be particularly poor; twenty- to thirty-nine-year-old female smokers ran twice as great a risk of being toothless or having advanced gum disease as did nonsmoking women their age. For men smokers, the comparable age range was thirty to fifty-nine.

Systemic diseases such as diabetes, certain blood disorders, and nutritional deficiencies increase the tendency of the periodontal tissue to break down. (On many occasions an alert dentist may note possible signs of early diabetes in a patient, who is then urged to check with a physician.) But since pyorrhea is usually caused by factors in the mouth, a dentist's major effort in therapy is usually to correct the local and more obvious conditions. The dentist uses special instruments to remove calculus from the necks of the teeth and from the periodontal pocket, and then smooths the tooth root. Any extensively damaged gingival tissue may have to be removed surgically.

After this treatment, the dentist may attack other causative factors. Abnormal occlusion can often be corrected by recontouring areas of the teeth to distribute pressure evenly. Missing teeth should, of course, be replaced promptly by bridgework to prevent drifting. If need be, the teeth in the dental arch can be completely rebuilt. (Even in early childhood, the premature loss of a baby molar deserves attention. A dentist may use space-maintenance techniques to prevent permanent teeth from erupting into faulty positions.)

BRUSHING AND FLOSSING

The major responsibility for the maintenance of healthy teeth and gums and the prevention of periodontal disease and tooth decay lies with the patient — not the dentist. A regimen for continuous plaque control is essential. According to CU's dental consultants, proper brushing and *daily flossing* (see page 73) are needed to prevent the buildup of plaque.

The first rule in dental care is cleanliness. An electric toothbrush can help some people (primarily the handicapped), but CU's dental consultants say that a powered brush in no way cleans teeth better than a *properly used* manual brush. For those, however, who feel they do a less-than-adequate job of manual brushing and may wish to consider an electric toothbrush, CU recommends that consideration be limited to models approved by the ADA. The ADA's Council on Dental Materials and Devices recognizes those models whose manufacturers have submitted valid clinical evidence that a brush provides "a high degree of oral cleanliness" and does not harm oral tissues.

But for most people the hand brush remains the preferred instrument. And those who wear braces may find electric brushes a nuisance (the bristles may become caught in the wires). In selecting a manual brush, choose a *soft* nylon brush with rounded bristles, one with a head that fits your mouth. There is, of course, a vast array of brushes on the market. The brush design you choose should depend in large part on the brushing technique you use. Therefore, consult with your dentist who can outline an efficient technique for manual brushing and recommend the kind of brush to buy. You may wish to refer to the booklet put out by the American Academy of Periodontology (see page 73) for a good description of a brushing technique. When a soft-bristle brush is used correctly — at least once a day for two to four minutes with proper brushing technique — it will wear enough to warrant replacement after about six weeks.

With proper brushing and flossing, once-a-day brushing should be sufficient. CU's dental consultants point out that brushing after every meal can't hurt, but that it is probably not necessary if plaque is properly removed once a day. Those over twenty-five may derive even more benefits from the mechanical action of a properly used brush than from any chemical supplied by a dentifrice. The brushing action removes the mat of plaque (and pellicle, its precursor), which constantly forms on teeth. But in acting against plaque, the brush can be helped by an appropriately formulated dentifrice. To that end, almost all dentifrices contain abrasives and, usually, a soap or detergent. Disclosing agents (tablets or liquids available from the dentist or drugstore) stain the plaque and highlight the areas most in need of persistent brushing.

As a matter of fact, many people do not do a reasonable job of brushing without a dentifrice containing at least some abrasive. If the abrasive is unduly harsh, however, brushers with receded gums are apt to damage the very teeth they are trying to preserve. Exposed root areas are especially sensitive to abrasion. With abrasion, a V-shaped notch is worn into the root of the tooth at the gum line, which weakens the crown of the tooth. For most people, then, *low-to-mild* abrasion is a good thing in regular brushing. But harsh abrasion is never recommended — even for those whose teeth are prone to staining. You are better off with stain than with excessive abrasion; when in doubt, consult your dentist.

In 1972 CU tested thirty-two toothpastes and one powder for their abrasiveness. The first concern of those conducting the tests was the effect of abrasion on enamel, the extremely hard material that sheaths all exposed tooth surfaces in a healthy mouth. No tested dentifrice was judged unduly harsh on enamel, and the differences that did emerge were so slight that they were not significant.

However, the effects on dentin (the inner, principal mass of a tooth), and the likely effects on cementum (the bony material that normally sheaths tooth areas below the gum), had more serious implications. (Although no tests were conducted on cementum, the dentin results were judged applicable to cementum.) Both those materials are considerably softer than enamel. Furthermore, they are apt to be exposed as the gums recede with age. About 15 percent of the population has exposed root surfaces by the age of twenty-nine; that figure rises to about 60 percent by the time people are in their fifties. Adverse effects of an unduly harsh abrasive on such susceptible surfaces are, of course, aggravated by any overenthusiasm with a toothbrush. Accordingly, CU made dentin abrasion the main consideration in its tests.

The original ADA-accepted fluoride pastes (*Colgate MFP*, *Crest Mint*, and *Crest Regular*) turned out to be considerably more abrasive than some of the other pastes. But manual brushers over twenty-five (with sound gums and no plastic bridgework) might still choose them, since there are at least some laboratory indications that fluoride might inhibit caries even in adults. Should irritation or taste problems crop up, *Gleem II* appeared to be a reasonable alternative; CU's tests suggested it had some potential for inhibiting decay, and it was an above-average cleaner and polisher.

Toothpastes may have an adverse effect on the gums of a small percentage of people; sensitivity to some elements of a paste's formulation could cause the gums to become shredded or sore. This kind of problem can often be cleared up by switching toothpaste brands.

People with gum troubles, those who use an electric tooth-brush, and those with fixed plastic crowns should always choose a less abrasive toothpaste. CU's tests indicated that *Pepsodent* and *Craig-Martin* were relatively gentle products. But removable dentures should not be brushed with any of the products tested by CU; the least risky cleaner for them is a soak-type product (see page 75).

A word now about the cosmetic effects of dentifrices on your teeth: To the degree that ad puffery about "whitening" and "brightening" means anything at all, it seems to relate almost exclusively to the incorporation of one or another of the harsher abrasives into a paste. The ADA has said it sees no valid reason for the use of a dentifrice with greater abrasiveness than would be necessary to prevent accumulation of plaque on the teeth.

Some toothpastes have used chloroform for flavoring because of its astringent or "biting" effect. The ADA reported in 1974 that *Ultra-Brite* and *Macleans* still included chloroform; *Close-Up* had already dropped the drug from its formulation. After studies showed that chloroform was cancer-causing in animals, the FDA in July 1976 banned the use of chloroform in drug and cosmetic products, including toothpastes. Because the FDA did not also recall existing products, the ban did not affect inventories on the shelves. The ADA reports, however, that chloroform had been removed from both *Macleans* and *Ultra-Brite* several months prior to the FDA's action against the drug. (CU's dental and medical consultants had questioned the need for including such an agent in dentifrices and are gratified that the FDA finally acted to prohibit use of chloroform in tooth-pastes.)

Ads for *Close-up*, *Vote*, *Pearl Drops*, and *Macleans* notwith-standing, none of the tested dentifrices contained whitening ingredients, bleaches, or anything else that can in any way alter the natural color of your teeth. You *can* brighten teeth — that is, heighten their luster somewhat — by polishing them. But all the more effective polishers among the tested products were also among the more abrasive. The Federal Trade Commission (FTC) has called on several dentifrice makers to substantiate ad claims dealing with whitening, abrasion, breath-freshening, cavity reduction, and the like. *Macleans*, for instance, was asked to justify advertising its paste as falling into the lowest third of all pastes in terms of abrasion, a statement CU's study certainly did not support. As of this writing the FTC reports that no further steps are planned against the *Macleans* advertisements.

Some other special situations deserve comment. Both *Thermodent* and *Sensodyne* have been promoted for "sensitive teeth." But the ADA's Council on Dental Therapeutics says it has not seen adequate evidence to justify any such claim. It is worth noting, though, that *Thermodent* was among the least abrasive of the products tested by CU, while *Sensodyne* was not. *Thermodent*, however, contains formaldehyde; CU questioned its safety in the mouth and stomach. *Extar* has been touted as helpful in removing calculus from teeth and retarding new calculus formation. The ADA, again, was unconvinced.

One recent caution in the selection of toothpastes can now be all but forgotten. In 1972 and 1973 studies reported that most brands of toothpaste contained lead, some in potentially hazardous amounts, in the outer coatings of the tube, the tube, and the paste itself. One report stated that of eighteen brands tested only two — *Binaca* and *Thermodent* — were completely lead-free. Fortunately, most manufacturers of dentifrices have since switched to nonlead containers and have thus largely eliminated the problem. A representative of the ADA's Council on Dental Therapeutics has reported to CU that at least 97 percent of all toothpastes are now marketed in nonlead containers, and an FDA spokesman agrees that the agency no longer considers this a problem. CU's medical and dental consultants believe that all toothpastes packaged in lead-containing tubes should be removed from the market and that the use of lead in toothpaste containers should be prohibited.

Brushing your teeth is only part of a well-rounded program of oral hygiene. A properly used brush can do a good job in removing the bacterial plaque that clings to teeth, but it is apt to miss plaque and food debris nestled in some areas between the teeth. So after you brush, it is important to use dental floss to clean between the teeth.

The American Academy of Periodontology recommends the following procedure: Cut off a long piece of floss, and lightly wrap the ends around your middle fingers. Insert the floss between each tooth and, holding it taut, move it gently back and forth past the point where the teeth contact each other. Move the floss with both fingers up and down five or six times on the side of one tooth, going down to the gum line but not into the gum. Repeat on the side of the adjacent tooth. When the floss becomes frayed or soiled, a turn around one middle finger brings up a fresh section. When you have done all your teeth, rinse vigorously with water (and do that, too, after eating, should you be unable to floss). Some dentists believe that unwaxed floss is better than waxed — CU suggests you ask your dentist for a recommendation. The American Academy of Periodontology booklet, "Effective Oral Hygiene," gives suggested techniques for brushing and flossing. It is available for 25¢ from AAP, Room 924, 211 East Chicago Avenue, Chicago, Illinois 60611.

A toothpick is never an adequate alternative to dental floss because it cannot reach into tight areas between teeth. Some dentists, however, suggest a specially shaped toothpick, such as the *Stim-u-dent*, or a brush equipped with a rubber interdental tip, because of the possible benefits from stimulation of the gums. If you wish to use a toothpick for removal of material from the mouth, CU's dental consultants recommend that you use it with a special toothpick holder, an inexpensive item available at a drugstore. The holder enables the toothpick to reach many areas of the mouth. Never pick the teeth with wires, pins, or matchbook covers, which can injure the gum between the teeth.

For some of their patients many dentists recommend the use of a dental irrigator as an adjunct to brushing and flossing. Basically, this device releases a fine stream of water at a fairly high pressure; the user directs the water toward, around, and between the teeth. The idea is to dislodge any food particles that brushing would not remove. This process can remove some of the irritants present in the mouth, but *not plaque*. Those who use a dental irrigator should direct the stream horizontally, rather than vertically, to avoid forcing debris into gum pockets or under gum flaps. Some dentists believe that at first you should set the pressure low and gradually increase it over days or weeks, instead of starting out with the highest pressure. In any event, a dental irrigator should be considered supplementary to regular oral hygiene. It is *not* a substitute for normal brushing and use of dental floss.

People with poorly controlled diabetes or chronic rheumatic heart disease should consult both their dentist and their physician before using a dental irrigator. However, a dental irrigator could be of particular benefit for those who wear braces or permanent bridgework. If your dentist has indicated that you should use a dental irrigator, limit your consideration to models that have been judged by the ADA to be safe for unsupervised use. However, CU tests in 1971 showed that only two of the four ADA-approved electric irrigators in the test were free from shock hazard (even when immersed in water). They were the *Water Pik 52* and the *General Electric AP2*. (The latter was discontinued in January 1974.)

Dental irrigators that attach directly to a faucet do basically the same thing as electric irrigators. And faucet irrigators are a lot simpler and less expensive. With no pump and no water reservoir, the faucet models are also more compact than most electric models. Yet they can have their problems too. An adapter must be attached to the faucet, and not all sinks come with faucets that are adaptable. The faucet models cannot be used with separate faucets for hot and cold water and are not recommended for use in homes subject to very high water pressure. CU's tests classified as acceptable the *Hydro Dent OH3*, with slightly lower ratings for the *Dento Spray MA* and the *Pulsar 70*.

Contrary to much advertising, chewing gum does not provide health benefits to the gums. Hard, fibrous foods (salads and raw fruits) produce a natural cleansing effect, but chewing gum does not. And it can aggravate the stresses and inflammation that go with pyorrhea. Moreover, the sugar in chewing gum — except for the "sugar-free" kind — promotes dental decay.

DENTURES

Of the soak-type denture products CU tested in 1971, CU recommended *Polident* tablets (or powder) for maintaining clean dentures. Soiled dentures, however, may benefit from use of *Denalan Denture Cleanser* (next-best choice: *Kleenite Denture Cleanser*) until the dentures are clean; after that, switch to *Polident*. CU's dental consultants were not impressed with the use of plain baking soda for cleansing dentures. And they strongly caution against the use of laundry bleach. Some additional words of advice to denture wearers: If possible, rinse your dentures after every meal; and when you are not wearing them, store them in a cleansing solution (or at least in water).

CU's dental consultants remind denture wearers that regular dental examinations are still essential. Loss of teeth in no way diminishes the need. The dentist will include a check on how the dentures fit and will examine for oral cancer and precancerous lesions.

Chapter 6

"Tired eyes" and eyewashes

AMONG THE LEAST USEFUL over-the-counter (OTC) remedies are the eyewashes, such as *Murine, Eye-Gene,* and *Visine*. *Eye-Gene* advertises: "Clears red eyes fast. Feel it soothe and refresh tired eyes too." This is a typical eyewash claim.

Although OTC eyewashes can produce a slight, brief, soothing effect, that is just about all that can be said for them. The fact is that normal eyes do not need cleansing, soothing, or refreshing by solutions of astringent and antiseptic chemicals. Simple irritation disappears of its own accord in about a day. No synthetic solution can match natural tears for washing away small bits of dust, dirt, and irritating material. And human tears contain an enzyme that has mild antibacterial properties at least as effective as those of the commercial eyewashes.

But essential uselessness is not the only criticism to be made of eyewashes. A more important fault is that their use may lead to the neglect of symptoms that indicate serious trouble. One of the most severe disorders that eye discomfort may signal is glaucoma. It is estimated that in the United States more than 1,700,000 people over thirty-five have this disease, and about 14 percent of all blindness is caused by it.

Glaucoma is an eye disease (the cause of which remains unknown) manifested by an increase in pressure within the eyeball. The elevated pressure then proceeds to affect the visual apparatus of the eye, leading in some cases to blindness. In closed-angle (acute) glaucoma, the eye becomes red and painful and usually requires emergency treatment by an ophthalmologist.

Some medications may precipitate a first attack of closed-angle glaucoma in people who are predisposed to the disease, often without being aware of their susceptibility. Such medications include antihistamines, which may be present in preparations used for the relief of colds (see Chapter 2) or for motion sickness, belladonna-type drugs sometimes taken for gastrointestinal disorders, OTC sleep remedies (see Chapter 24), and tricyclic antidepressants (see Chapter 25). Because of its sudden onset, such an attack is not likely to be neglected. But in simple (chronic) glaucoma the only complaint may be indefinite eye discomfort without redness — precisely the kind of discomfort for which some people may use OTC remedies.

Many people have simple glaucoma without knowing it, and the disease can do irreparable damage to the sight without ever causing marked discomfort. Because of the prevalence of glaucoma in the adult population, the National Society for the Prevention of Blindness, and practicing eye specialists as well, urge glaucoma screening tests during periodic health checkups for adults over thirty-five (sooner for diabetics). If detected early, glaucoma can be treated — and sight saved. When you have your next eye checkup, it may be wise to ask the ophthalmologist or optometrist whether you are susceptible to closed-angle glaucoma and thus should be wary of using the above-mentioned drugs.

Smarting, burning, itching, and inflammation of the whites of the eye (conjunctivitis) and eyelids (blepharitis) are often caused by infection with bacteria or viruses or by allergic sensitivity to dust, pollens, or molds. Most bacterial infections of the eyes can be cured fairly quickly by antibiotic drops or ointments prescribed by a physician. Authorities now believe that viral infections of the eyes occur more frequently than previously supposed. Conjunctivitis, often referred to as "pink eye," frequently occurs a few days after bathing in a swimming pool, even an adequately chlorinated pool. The discomfort may be severe. The infection usually requires a visit to a physician for proper diagnosis and treatment.

An acute inflammatory disorder of the eyes may in reality be a localized manifestation of a systemic infection. Reddening of the eyes and sensitivity to light are common with measles. It is not unusual for mild inflammation of the eyes to accompany viral respiratory infections, especially those caused by adenovirus. Chronic inflammation of certain parts of the eye may signal the onset of a general disease, such as rheumatoid arthritis or sarcoidosis.

Eye fatigue may result from errors of refraction, such as astigmatism, farsightedness, or nearsightedness; it may be associated with general fatigue, such as that resulting from a sleepless night. There are various systemic diseases, such as hyperthyroidism or myasthenia gravis, that affect the eye muscles and lids, giving rise to so-called eye fatigue.

It is apparent from this brief catalog of the possible causes of common eye complaints that they cannot be effectively treated with OTC solutions. If any of these symptoms persists more than a day or so, the eyes should be examined by a physician. Then, if the doctor gives them a clean bill of health and you still want an eyewash to relieve simple irritation caused by smog, strong light, sea bathing, or bathing in chlorinated water, one or two drops of cold tap water, placed in the lower lid with a clean eye dropper, should be adequate. The same treatment, or the application of iced wet compresses for about fifteen minutes, safely relieves "tired" though otherwise healthy eyes.

CU's medical consultants believe that a boric acid solution should never be used as an eyewash because of possible toxicity (see page 311). Furthermore, such solutions have not been shown to be more effective than plain water for the relief of eye discomfort.

Beyond any claimed therapeutic effect, some of the OTC eye solutions seem to offer a cosmetic benefit: "Get the red out," says one ad. A topical vasoconstrictor (such as tetrahydrozoline in *Visine*) should not be used regularly for cosmetic purposes. Such use risks a rebound effect in which the condition returns with increasing severity which would then require increasing frequency of dosage.

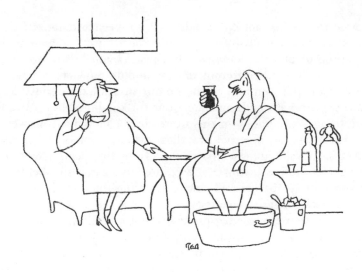

"To the common cold!"

Chapter 7

Indigestion and antacids

OVER THE YEARS, antacid products have been promoted for a host of common ills — from simple "heartburn" or mild indigestion, to bloating, cramps, "gas pains," and "morning sickness." At least 575 different tablets, liquids, powders, lozenges, gums, and pills compete to soothe our stomach complaints. Yet fewer than a dozen brands account for the lion's share of advertising — and sales — in this more than $200 million market.

How safe or effective are these widely promoted brands? And how valid are the advertising claims for them? Exact answers are elusive, because "indigestion" is a catch-all label for a variety of symptoms, and tests comparing the touted remedies often lack scientific validity.

Indigestion can be a temporary symptom following an elaborate meal, or a recurrent symptom signaling a more serious problem, such as a peptic ulcer. It may result directly from one of several diseases of the upper digestive tract, or it may be a sign of another disorder, such as motion sickness or heart disease. In fact, heart disease is one of the most important causes of indigestionlike symptoms in middle-aged men. Indigestion may also be a side effect of many prescription drugs, particularly antibiotics, as well as cortisone and other anti-arthritis medicines. Such symptoms can usually be alleviated by taking the medication on a full stomach or with milk, although this procedure may lessen the effectiveness of certain antibiotics by reducing absorption. (When in doubt, consult your pharmacist or physician.)

The occasional digestive upset that follows overindulgence, a rough day at the office, or a family squabble is usually no cause for alarm, and may be treated with a variety of familiar remedies, including ordinary baking soda. But there are three situations that call for immediate medical attention: any single episode of severe or persistent discomfort, especially if accompanied by sweating, weakness, or breathlessness; any single episode accompanied by vomiting of blood; and repeated episodes of indigestion — no matter how mild. "Repeated" may mean as infrequently as a few times a month for several months. In such instances, self-medication with an antacid can be dangerous, because it may mask a serious disorder and thus delay essential medical treatment.

Even in illnesses in which antacids are an accepted part of therapy — such as peptic ulcer — self-medication without medical supervision can be extremely hazardous. Although a physician may prescribe an antacid for the temporary relief of ulcer pain, the ulcer may still become worse and the patient must be closely observed. If perforation should occur, leakage of gastric or intestinal contents could cause intense pain, infection, shock, and even death.

In short, indiscriminate use of antacids can involve real perils — a fact that is rarely, if ever, noted in the ads for these nonprescription items.

One of the oldest and most familiar antacids is sodium bicarbonate, or common baking soda. It is currently a major ingredient of *Alka-Seltzer* and *Bromo Seltzer* — the two top sellers in the antacid field — and of several lesser known brands including *Bell-Ans, Brioschi, Eno,* and *Fizrin.* Sodium bicarbonate is a potent and fast-acting antacid, but one of the least desirable for regular or frequent use. If taken daily for more than a few weeks by people with diminished kidney function, a bicarbonate-containing antacid may disturb the body's acid-base balance and cause the body fluids to become more alkaline than normal. Prolonged use of such an alkalinizing agent may even lead to kidney stone formation and may also contribute to recurrent urinary tract infections.

What's more, the large amounts of sodium in *Alka-Seltzer* and *Bromo Seltzer* (see table on page 90) can be harmful to individuals with hypertension or congestive heart failure or to anyone else who must restrict sodium intake for whatever reason. For example, a heart patient allowed only 1,000 to 2,000 milligrams of sodium daily would risk upsetting that regimen with a single dose of *Alka-Seltzer* or *Bromo Seltzer*. In a customary two-tablet dose, *Alka-Seltzer* contains 1,042 milligrams of sodium. *Bromo Seltzer* has 748 milligrams per capful. (The recommended dose of *Bromo Seltzer* is "one or two heaping capfuls.") In short, because of hazards associated with both sodium and bicarbonate, antacids containing sodium bicarbonate should be strictly limited to healthy individuals — and only for occasional use.

The Food and Drug Administration (FDA) panel on antacids, which published its report in April 1973, judged unsuitable for people on low-salt diets any antacid containing more than 115 milligrams of sodium per maximum daily use. Since many people have undetected heart or kidney disorders and the prevalence of these conditions increases with age, the panel recommended that no more than 2,300 milligrams of sodium per day in antacids be taken by *anyone* over sixty years of age. Yet the maximum daily dosages suggested on current labels of *Alka-Seltzer* (eight tablets) and *Bromo Seltzer* (six capfuls) contain more than the recommended safe amount of sodium.

In addition to their high sodium content, *Alka-Seltzer* and *Bromo Seltzer* also contain large amounts of citrates. A maximum daily dose of eight *Alka-Seltzer* tablets, or more than three capfuls of *Bromo Seltzer*, exceeds the safe limits for citrates (8 grams) recommended by the FDA panel.

Another serious disadvantage of *Alka-Seltzer* for regular use as an antacid is its aspirin content, which can be dangerous in an antacid, especially if the symptoms stem from ulcers or other serious stomach disorders (see Chapter 1). The FDA panel concluded that antacid/aspirin combinations "are irrational for antacid use alone and therefore should not be labeled or marketed for such use." However, the occasional use of an antacid/aspirin combination to relieve the discomfort of a combined headache and upset stomach seems reasonable. But *repeated* use for treatment of this double affliction, or for relief of either set of symptoms, is not recommended by CU's medical consultants.

Over the years, CU's medical consultants have frequently advised against the regular use of *Alka-Seltzer* as an antacid. In their judgment, its continued popularity is a clear defeat for public health education. However, the findings of the FDA panel — and perhaps the possibility of government intervention — appear to have influenced advertising for *Alka-Seltzer*. As of this writing, the product is being promoted for those suffering simultaneously from headache and stomach upset who may wish to avoid taking both ordinary aspirin and a simple antacid. This theme may make more medical sense but, CU believes, the advertising should also include information about the hazards of repeated dosage.*

While *Bromo Seltzer* trails well behind *Alka-Seltzer* in advertising and sales, it runs neck and neck in dubious safety

---

* In 1974, Miles Laboratories, the makers of *Alka-Seltzer*, began nationwide distribution of a new product, *Alka-Seltzer Without Aspirin*. According to the manufacturer, the only change in formulation was the elimination of *Alka-Seltzer*'s aspirin content. In 1975, Miles introduced a chewable product, *Alka-2*, containing calcium carbonate (see page 85).

credentials. Like *Alka-Seltzer, Bromo Seltzer* adds analgesics to a potent dose of antacid. Although its analgesics — acetaminophen and phenacetin — do not irritate the stomach as aspirin does, they are also unnecessary in an antacid. And phenacetin, now banned in Canada for certain uses, has been associated with kidney damage in long-term users (see page 17). Furthermore, *Bromo Seltzer* also contains approximately 32.5 milligrams of caffeine per capful — or about as much as a quarter cup of brewed coffee. Caffeine stimulates acid secretion in the stomach and is therefore inappropriate for ulcer patients. Its presence in an antacid is no more justifiable than that of aspirin. In short, instead of the aspirin used in *Alka-Seltzer, Bromo Seltzer* substitutes two other analgesics which are unnecessary in an antacid, and a stimulant which should not be there at all.

In the judgment of CU's medical consultants, ordinary sodium bicarbonate neutralizes stomach acid as adequately as any of the costlier products containing it. People who would rather take an effervescent product, however, should be careful to choose one that is basically a straight antacid. Such products as *Brioschi* and *Eno*, for example, contain no other active ingredients than antacids. Both are high in sodium bicarbonate, however, and consequently should *not* be used regularly or frequently by healthy people, or be used at all by those on low-salt diets (see page 82). *Fizrin*, which contains aspirin and is generally similar in composition to *Alka-Seltzer*, also contains sodium carbonate (not bicarbonate). *The Pharmacological Basis of Therapeutics*, edited by Drs. Louis S. Goodman and Alfred Gilman, reports that sodium carbonate "is obsolete as an antacid because it is highly alkaline and irritating, and can even be corrosive." Accordingly, CU's medical consultants judge *Fizrin* to be an even worse choice for use as a regular antacid.

Until a few years ago, calcium carbonate prescribed in

powder form was the antacid of choice among many physicians; it provided rapid action and a high neutralizing capacity. Calcium carbonate is still the principal antacid in numerous over-the-counter products, including *Tums* and *Pepto-Bismol* tablets (but not *Pepto-Bismol* liquid; see page 86). However, this compound tends to cause constipation; and, more seriously, its prolonged use may raise calcium in the blood to undesirable levels and cause impaired kidney function and possible stone formation. The likelihood of developing high blood calcium levels appears to increase for those who frequently consume large amounts of milk or who have kidney problems to begin with.

To prevent harmful effects, the FDA antacid panel advised against taking more than 8 grams of calcium carbonate daily. Labeling proposed by the panel would also limit this dosage level to a maximum period of two weeks, "except under the advice and supervision of a physician." Currently, each *Tums* tablet contains approximately ½ gram of calcium carbonate, while a *Pepto-Bismol* tablet contains about ⅓ gram. Thus the maximum daily dosage of *Tums*, for example, should not exceed sixteen tablets, nor should use at this level extend beyond two weeks. The experience of CU's medical consultants indicates that many current users exceed these amounts.

Recent research suggests that calcium carbonate can cause an "acid rebound." A study published in *The New England Journal of Medicine* in September 1973 indicated that significant increases in stomach acid production followed the ingestion by healthy individuals of as little as ½ gram of calcium carbonate. (Some of the brands whose recommended single dosage contains approximately ½ gram or more of calcium carbonate include *Alkets, Camalox, Dicarbosil, Ducon, Titralac* liquid, and *Tums*.) Although the mechanism of this stomach acid release is unknown, that same study showed mild elevations in blood levels of gastrin, a hormone produced in the stomach and known to facilitate secretion of acid by the stomach. Consequently, the effect of antacids containing calcium may be self-defeating. More work remains to be done on this question, however. Meanwhile, CU's medical consultants advise against the routine use of antacids containing calcium carbonate, particularly those with significant amounts in the formulation.

Tums and *Rolaids* are both available in convenient roll packs, but there the similarity ends. In contrast to *Tums'* main antacid ingredient, calcium carbonate, *Rolaids* contains an antacid that combines sodium bicarbonate and aluminum hydroxide (see below). While *Tums* is low in sodium, *Rolaids* contains 53 milligrams of it per tablet — which is high for anyone who must restrict salt intake. Occasional use of either *Tums* or *Rolaids* presents little hazard. However, because of the calcium content of *Tums* and the sodium bicarbonate properties of *Rolaids*, neither product is suitable for frequent, long-term use.

Label claims for *Pepto-Bismol* liquid and tablets may lead a buyer to think that both forms of the product are much the same. However, a closer look at the labels reveals that while the tablets contain two antacids — calcium carbonate and glycocoll — the liquid has none at all, despite label claims that it relieves indigestion. Indeed, *Pepto-Bismol* liquid is not an antacid, but rather an aid "for digestive upsets" — whatever that means. The liquid contains bismuth subsalicylate as its main ingredient. Goodman and Gilman's *The Pharmacological Basis of Therapeutics* observes: "Inefficacy and toxic potential have led to the gradual disuse of bismuth preparations, although they are still exploited commercially." What's more, those taking the tablets for acid indigestion may get more than they bargain for, since the calcium carbonate included in the tablets has a constipating effect. In view of potential side effects, including possible darkening of the tongue and blackening of the stools (which may mask gastrointestinal bleeding from an ulcer), CU's medical consultants advise against the use of *Pepto-Bismol* products.

In contrast to its warnings on bicarbonate, calcium, citrates, and sodium, the FDA panel found two other common antacid ingredients to be relatively nonhazardous. It judged aluminum compounds to be safe in the amounts usually taken, and placed no dosage restrictions on them. It reached a similar verdict on magnesium compounds, except for patients with chronic kidney diseases. Since these patients have less ability to eliminate magnesium from their bodies, the panel set a dosage limit in such cases.

The best known aluminum compound is aluminum hydroxide. *Amphojel* is one of the few examples of an antacid using aluminum hydroxide as its single ingredient. Although its onset of effect is slow and its neutralizing capacity variable, aluminum hydroxide provides relatively prolonged antacid action. Aluminum compounds also decrease the absorption of phosphate in the intestine, an effect that may benefit kidney patients who have elevated blood phosphate levels. However, aluminum compounds may cause severe constipation, which has tended to limit the popularity of products depending on this antacid ingredient alone. To offset the drawback, aluminum hydroxide is often combined with magnesium compounds, which tend to have a laxative effect. (For a discussion of magnesium/aluminum products, see below.)

Magnesium hydroxide may be purchased as milk of magnesia, a simple antacid available under this generic name at any pharmacy. The main ingredient in any brand of milk of magnesia, magnesium hydroxide, is an effective and generally safe antacid. The problem with such products, however, is their laxative effect. Ordinarily, the antacid dosage of, for example, *Phillips' Milk of Magnesia* is one to three teaspoons (or two to four tablets). The same product is advertised as a laxative at a dosage of two to four tablespoons (or six to eight tablets).

Consequently, people who repeat the antacid dosage or who are more susceptible than others to its laxative action may experience an unwanted side effect.

People with chronic kidney disorders should not use milk of magnesia or other magnesium antacids on a regular basis except under the supervision of a physician. More than three teaspoons (or more than four tablets) per day of *Phillips' Milk of Magnesia* exceeds the safe limit for magnesium set by the FDA panel for chronic kidney patients.

CU's medical consultants believe that the antacid products most likely to offer relative safety and a minimum of side effects — particularly for long-term use — are those containing aluminum hydroxide and magnesium hydroxide or trisilicate. Products containing both aluminum hydroxide and magnesium hydroxide include *Aludrox, Creamalin, Maalox, Magnesium-Aluminum Hydroxide Gel USP, Maxamag Suspension*, and *WinGel*. These brands are available in either liquid or suspension formulation. In addition to employing aluminum and magnesium hydroxides together, *Di-Gel* and *Mylanta* contain simethicone (an antiflatulent, not an antacid), which the manufacturers say may help to relieve "gas pains."

Of the products combining magnesium trisilicate with aluminum hydroxide, *Gelusil* is the most familiar. As in aluminum compounds, the antacid action of magnesium trisilicate is slow in onset but is of comparatively long duration. Other brands with this combination include *A.M.T.*, *Malcogel*, and *Trisogel*. (These products, too, can be obtained in either liquid or suspension formulation.)

A study in *The New England Journal of Medicine*, published in May 1973, reported that products with magnesium hydroxide are faster in onset of action and higher in acid-neutralizing capacity than those with magnesium trisilicate. Both compounds, however, were judged potentially effective by the FDA panel. A few products, such as *Magnatril* and

Mucotin, apparently "just to be sure," combine aluminum hydroxide with *both* magnesium hydroxide and trisilicate.

Among the most important findings of the FDA panel were its conclusions about product claims. The panel declared that antacids can relieve heartburn, sour stomach, or acid indigestion, but that any other claim is unfounded. Assertions that a product can alleviate nervous or emotional disturbances, "acidosis," "food intolerance," or morning sickness of pregnancy were found untruthful or inaccurate. Also judged unproven or unlikely were claims for relieving such symptoms as "gas," nausea, upset stomach, "full feeling," and the like. In short, the panel concluded that an antacid performs only one function: It neutralizes acid — period.

In addition to limiting label claims, the monograph prepared by the FDA panel on antacids lists the active ingredients the panel found to be safe and effective. For some of these ingredients the panel set the maximum amount to be allowed in an antacid product. Once published in final form, the monograph will have the force of law. Manufacturers of nonconforming antacid products will be given six months in which to comply with the regulations or to remove their products from the market.

Decisions by the panel about effective ingredients, dosage levels, product claims, and labeling should help you make a more rational selection of an antacid preparation. CU's medical consultants urge you to consider the following guidelines when you think you need an antacid:

■ Do not use any antacid regularly for more than several weeks, except with the advice and supervision of a physician.

■ Restrict sodium bicarbonate or calcium carbonate antacids to occasional use only, and give preference to products with aluminum and magnesium ingredients.

■ If you are on a sodium-restricted diet, stick to an antacid low in sodium. Check the table on page 90; if necessary, ask

Ingredients of selected antacid products

	Form	Major antacid
Alka-Seltzer	tablet	sodium bicarbonate
Bromo Seltzer	granules	sodium bicarbonate
Di-Gel	liquid	aluminum hydroxide, magnesium hydroxide
	tablet	aluminum hydroxide, magnesium hydroxide
Gelusil	liquid or tablet	aluminum hydroxide, magnesium trisilicate
Maalox	liquid or tablet	aluminum hydroxide, magnesium hydroxide
Mylanta	liquid or tablet	aluminum hydroxide, magnesium hydroxide
Pepto-Bismol	tablet‡	calcium carbonate§
Phillips' Milk of Magnesia	liquid or tablet	magnesium hydroxide
Rolaids	tablet	dihydroxyaluminum sodium carbonate
Tums	tablet	calcium carbonate§

* Antacids with more than 115 mg of sodium per maximum daily dose should not be used by patients on low-salt diets, except with the advice and supervision of a physician. In general, products containing 9 mg or less per normal dose are preferred for such use.

† *Maalox No. 1* contains 1 mg of sodium per tablet; *Maalox No. 2* contains 2 mg.

Other antacid	Nonantacid	Approximate sodium content in milligrams (mg)°
citric acid, monocalcium phosphate	aspirin	521 mg per tablet
citric acid	acetaminophen, caffeine, phenacetin	748 mg per capful
—	simethicone	9 mg per teaspoon
magnesium carbonate	simethicone	9 mg per tablet
—	—	7 mg per teaspoon; 5 mg per tablet
—	—	6 mg per teaspoon; 1 or 2 mg per tablet†
—	simethicone	4 mg per teaspoon; 1 mg per tablet
glycocoll	bismuth subsalicylate	less than 1 mg per tablet
—	—	1 mg per teaspoon; 2.5 mg per tablet
—	—	53 mg per tablet
magnesium carbonate, magnesium trisilicate	—	3 mg per tablet

‡ The liquid form of *Pepto-Bismol* is not an antacid.

§ Note text on page 85.

Sources: Product label; product manufacturer; *Handbook of Non-Prescription Drugs*, 1973 edition, American Pharmaceutical Association; *The Medical Letter*, April 13, 1973. Sodium content of *Bromo Seltzer* is estimated from product ingredients.

your pharmacist or physician for a recommendation.

▪ The liquid or suspension form of an antacid seems to be more effective than the equivalent dose in tablets. To be effective tablets must be thoroughly sucked or chewed; otherwise they may not dissolve completely in the stomach before being discharged into the small intestine.

▪ If a certain food or beverage consistently causes stomach upsets, it makes more sense to cut out the troublemaker than to resort to medicine to relieve the symptoms. Should you fail to identify the culprit in your diet that is the probable cause of abdominal discomfort, or should you be uncertain, it may be wise to seek medical advice.

▪ And most important, if repeated or painful episodes of indigestion occur, stop self-medication and self-diagnosis and consult your physician.

▪ A special word for women who are pregnant: Because pregnant women must be careful to restrict aspirin intake for several weeks before the expected delivery date (see page 24), they should shun antacid preparations containing aspirin. They should also be cautious about frequent use of antacids with a high sodium content. Although it has now been shown that sodium is not generally harmful to pregnant women and, in fact, does not increase the hazard of toxemia, the ingestion of excessive amounts of sodium is a practice that would be sanctioned by few, if any, obstetricians. CU's medical consultants urge pregnant women to check with their doctors before taking any antacid preparations to relieve symptoms of stomach distress — and for that matter before taking *any* drug (see Chapter 23).

Chapter 8

Constipation and diarrhea

MOST CASES OF CONSTIPATION cure themselves without the use of drugs, although there are circumstances in which a mild laxative can be beneficial and relatively harmless. When, for example, there is temporary difficulty in evacuation due to emotional stress, traveling, or change in diet, there is no harm in taking a mild laxative for a day or two. And in some cases of chronic constipation – if it has definitely been proved to exist and there is no organic cause – a physician may suggest a laxative to help relieve the condition. But the widespread overdependence on laxatives, which supports the sale of more than 700 over-the-counter (OTC) laxative products, can be explained only by an equally widespread misunderstanding of constipation and the drugs used to treat it.

There is no such thing as a perfect, natural, or entirely harmless laxative. All types have some disadvantages. Moreover, the distinction that the advertisers of commercial products make between mild laxatives and harsh cathartics is highly deceptive. *Any* material taken by mouth to promote evacuation of the intestine is a cathartic drug; a laxative is simply a mild cathartic. But one person's laxative may be another's cathartic. Furthermore, in the same person a drug can act as a laxative at one time and a cathartic at another.

There can be no doubt that laxatives have contributed more to the ills and discomforts of mankind than the condition they are supposed to relieve. Instances of a ruptured appendix with peritonitis have been recorded in patients who assumed their abdominal pain was caused by constipation and so dosed themselves with laxatives. Constipation is rarely associated with severe abdominal pain. Nor does the presence of pain mean the bowels need to be cleaned out.

Who has not heard that, at the beginning of a cold or an attack of grippe, flu, or acute tonsilitis, a cathartic should be taken? This myth is a holdover from the Middle Ages when "a dose of the salts" was supposed to cure everything from ague to plague. Yet catharsis does not prevent, abort, or lessen the severity of these illnesses or any other acute illness. In acute illnesses, constipation may simply be associated with dehydration, poor intake of food, or prolonged inactivity. To purge a patient who is already suffering from depleted fluid reserves is foolish, and may even be disastrous.

No organ of the body is as misunderstood, maltreated, and fussed over as the digestive tract. It has been purged, irrigated, lavaged, massaged, and pummeled, all in the name of that great American obsession, the daily bowel movement. It is commonly believed that the waste matter left after digestion has been completed must be expelled twenty-four to forty-eight hours after the food is eaten. The fallacy of this impression was revealed in an experiment supervised by Dr. Walter C. Alvarez. A group of healthy young medical students swallowed sets of gelatin capsules containing many small glass beads. The results were interesting. Two of the students passed about 85 percent of the beads in twenty-four hours; most took four days to eliminate three-fourths of the beads; some passed only half of the beads in nine days.

Dr. Alvarez further observed that those who passed the majority of the beads in twenty-four hours had poorly formed stools containing undigested material. Those with a slower rate usually had well-formed stools showing evidence of good digestion. Some of the participants with the slower rates had believed that they were constipated.

Dr. Alvarez has likened the colon to a railroad siding on which three freight cars are standing. Every day a new car arrives and bumps the end one off, leaving three again. But occasionally one arrives at the siding with such force that it bumps all three off, and then three days must elapse before the siding is full again. In other words, when the colon is cleaned out by a purge or large bowel movement, nothing more should be expected for several days.

Nor does everyone operate on a once-a-day schedule. It is common to find people in perfect health who regularly defecate twice daily, and others who have an evacuation only once in two or three days without the slightest ill effect. There are many individuals who have regular bowel movements at still longer intervals without any impairment in health.

Constipation, then, cannot be defined in terms of a daily bowel movement, but must be related to each person's normal functioning. Missing a few bowel movements should cause no panic. After a few days, things generally return to normal, and the rhythm is reestablished.

When true chronic constipation is present, it may result from overemphasis on toilet training in childhood, irregular bowel habits, crowded living conditions, improper diet, or the like. A small percentage of patients with constipation have an organic disease such as diverticulitis or cancer. This cause is most likely to be found in adults who have previously had regular and satisfactory evacuation but then begin to experience a persistent change in the character or frequency of bowel movements. To investigate the possibility of organic disease, a doctor may directly observe the rectum and lower bowel through a lighted tube called a sigmoidoscope. The physician may also have a radiologist perform a barium-enema X-ray examination to inspect the remainder of the large bowel. But to repeat, constipation caused by an organic disease is not common. In general, if constipation has been present for years, the likelihood is that it is not due to serious disease.

More often, bowel dysfunction reflects emotional stresses. Such influences on the colon may be important, and also quite perverse. In one person they may speed up bowel transit time for ingested foodstuffs and cause diarrhea with occasional mucus in the stool. In another they may slow bowel activity and cause hard, dry, and infrequent stools. In a third they may lead to intestinal spasms perceived as painful abdominal cramps.

When these conditions recur or persist, they are known collectively as the irritable colon syndrome. This is the likely diagnosis in the case of long-standing bowel complaints associated with worry, fear, and anxiety. The irritable colon syndrome is an emotionally triggered disorder in which the intestine functions like a barometer. Irregular peristalsis not only results in abdominal pains and distention, but also in excessive passage of gas; and hard stools often alternate with looser stools. Treatment of the irritable colon syndrome calls for treatment of the underlying psychological disorder and whatever else serves to cushion anxiety and distress. (Bloody stools, which usually are not associated with the irritable colon syndrome, always require consultation with a physician.)

The irritable colon syndrome is no longer considered the only cause for complaints of bloating, gaseous distention, and intermittent loose stools. It has now been shown that for some people a more likely explanation may be what was formerly called an intestinal "allergy." A physician may discover through careful questioning that the discomfort is due to a food intolerance. One of the most frequent causes is the lack of an intestinal enzyme — lactase — which is essential for the proper digestion of milk products. These foods tend to precipitate episodes of abdominal discomfort. Similar patterns may follow ingestion of other foods, but the lactase deficiency syndrome has been the best studied thus far.

Unfortunately, the symptoms of an irritable colon, or even of lactase deficiency, are not always evident. For example, the emotional factors responsible for bowel dysfunction may not be obvious, so that it is not always possible for the sufferers to know that their constipation or diarrhea is of this type. This is another reason why proper diagnosis is important before a course of treatment for chronic constipation or diarrhea is begun.

Some medications frequently cause loose, watery bowel movements. The most common offenders include such antibiotics as lincomycin, ampicillin, and tetracycline. Also capable of provoking diarrhea are some magnesium-containing antacids (see page 87) and ascorbic acid (vitamin C).

If an attack of diarrhea does not subside in a day, or if diarrhea is accompanied at any time by fever, severe abdominal pain, or bloody stools, self-medication is not advisable, and the patient should consult a physician. In any case, a person suffering from diarrhea should drink plenty of liquids to offset loss of fluids in the watery stools. Decreasing the amount of roughage (or bulk producers) in the diet — for example, cutting out most raw fruits and raw vegetables — plus the time-honored reliance on rice and bananas may reduce the severity of the attack.

OTC preparations commonly used for acute diarrhea, such as kaolin/pectin mixtures (*Kaopectate*, *Paocin*, *Pektamalt*, among others), are less effective than antidiarrheal drugs containing codeine or opium. The latter are narcotic drugs, which require a prescription. Physicians may prescribe a small quantity of codeine tablets, tincture of opium, powdered opium in capsules, paregoric, or for adults the more expensive Lomotil — a tablet containing diphenoxylate (a synthetic narcotic).

These drugs are effective in relieving diarrhea reasonably promptly. In the amounts used for occasional diarrheal attacks, they should present no problem of dependency. CU's medical consultants warn against the use of Lomotil for infants and toddlers. Toxicity has been observed with minimal dosage.

The affliction commonly referred to as "acute gastro-enteritis" usually involves two or three days of diarrhea, along with fever and general malaise. This illness is now thought to be viral in origin. Healthy individuals are able to withstand such illnesses with only minor discomfort. However, the very young and the very old tend to fare less well. Because of the need for adequate fluid replacement, some may even require hospitalization.

Most attacks of diarrhea tend to be self-limited with the symptoms relieved (with or without medication) in a few days. However, diarrhea can be protracted, lasting more than a week. In the beginning stages underlying causes of protracted diarrhea such as amebic dysentery or ulcerative colitis may be difficult to diagnose. Since specific therapy for a disease must often await such diagnosis, it is important, when diarrhea is prolonged, to have microscopic and bacteriological examinations made of the stool, as well as sigmoidoscopic examination of the rectum. X rays of the bowel may also be necessary.

The cause of chronic constipation is frequently more prosaic, however. Something as simple as improper toilet habits may be an underlying cause. When the urge to defecate is disregarded, the sensation passes. It usually returns again during the day, especially after meals, but if the call is consistently disobeyed day after day, the rectum may eventually fail to signal the need for evacuation. The result may be severe constipation.

Why is the call disregarded? It may be suppressed, or it may be overwhelmed by other and stronger stimuli, similar to loss of one's appetite on hearing a piece of bad news. It may also be neglected because of the pressure of school or work, or perhaps because there is a morning train to catch or but one bathroom for a large family.

The misuse of laxatives is another important cause of chronic constipation. Whatever the original reason for starting it, repeated purgation in time brings changes in the lining and muscle tone of the bowel; the lining can become irritated and inflamed, and with long-continued catharsis muscular reflexes can become so diminished that stronger and stronger stimulation is required to produce any activity. Moreover, there are comparatively few users of cathartics who have not suffered from fissure of the anus or hemorrhoids (see Chapter 9). Such ailments often make defecation so painful that the sufferer tends to postpone a visit to the toilet, with the same results as those occurring in a person who is too busy. Chronic laxative users may also unknowingly be depleting their bodies of potassium, resulting in muscle weakness.

Of major importance as a possible cause of constipation are many OTC and prescription drugs in common use today. Antacids may often be a source of difficulty (see Chapter 7). Among the prescription drugs the most notorious offenders are narcotics such as opium, codeine, and oxycodone (the active ingredient in Percodan). Another class of compounds capable of causing constipation includes those affecting the parasympathetic nervous system. Among these drugs are antispasmodics such as propantheline (Pro-Banthine), antidepressants such as imipramine (Tofranil), and major tranquilizers such as chlorpromazine (Thorazine). Should constipation become severe after use of these drugs, a physician may decrease dosage or switch to another medication in order to relieve discomfort caused by the side effect.

Against this background of the cause — more properly, causes — of constipation, some rational approaches to treatment suggest themselves. If you think you have chronic constipation, the first thing to do is to stop taking laxatives. Many people who have done so at the insistence of a doctor have been surprised to find that, after a few days or a week, the bowels begin to move effectively again. For temporary constipation, the obvious thing to do is nothing; let nature take its course, and the condition will cure itself. But some people complain of headache or sluggishness or they just plain worry if they don't have a regular bowel movement; for such people it may be less harmful to use a laxative once in a while than to fret. The mildest laxative that produces results is the best choice (see page 102).

Some people may find it more natural, if not as convenient, to use an enema instead of a laxative. As authorities have been saying for many years, it does seem unreasonable to upset 25 feet of intestine with a cathartic when the trouble is in the last 8 inches — the rectum and anal canal. An enema consisting of a pint of tepid tap water is generally sufficient. While relatively expensive, prepackaged disposable enemas (e.g., *Fleet*) can be a convenience. But too frequent enemas — even once a week, for some people — can result in inability to initiate a bowel movement without recourse to an enema. (High colonic enemas, incidentally, are antiquated, useless, and sometimes harmful. They do not cure habitual constipation or remove "toxins," and in general do not promote health or prolong life.)

Glycerin suppositories have also been employed to stimulate evacuation of the rectum without disturbing the rest of the bowel. Their occasional use does no harm, but most physicians believe that for many individuals frequent use can cause irritation of the anus and mucous membrane of the rectum.

Without subscribing to the hysterics of food faddists, it would be an advantage to some people to add roughage (or bulk producers) to their diet in the form of fruits, vegetables, and whole-grain cereals. Among the more valuable foods for this purpose are bran, spinach, raw carrots, and whole fruit. Bran, often promoted for constipation, may be particularly useful for those who do not object to immediate and dramatic results. Cereals with the highest bran content include Kellogg's *All-Bran* and *Bran Buds*, and Post's and Kellogg's *40% Bran Flakes* and *Raisin Bran*. Prunes, the traditional friend of the constipated, provide bulk and stimulate peristalsis. Peristalsis may also be aided through use of prune extract or prune juice.

Remember, however, that the human intestinal tract is not constructed like that of a plant-eating animal. It is able to digest a wide variety of foods, but not the diet of a cow or rabbit. Also, there are individual idiosyncrasies. Some people can eat a high percentage of roughage without the slightest inconvenience. The same meal can produce distress in others. If pain, distention, mucus in the stool, or other evidence of irritation occurs, a physician should be consulted.

The role of exercise in the treatment of constipation has been exaggerated, but it may divert one's thoughts from working cares or household worries, thus conferring the sense of relaxation that facilitates a bowel movement. Massaging the abdominal muscles is a waste of time as therapy for constipation. And there is little value in drinking large quantities of water — even hot water flavored with lemon. However, any of these measures may have an important psychological effect.

If simple measures don't clear up constipation within a week or so, the trouble very likely is true chronic constipation, and a doctor's help is needed. Rational treatment must be based on the cause, and that can be established for sure only through a physical examination and careful questioning. A doctor takes daily living habits and diet into account. Often a laxative is prescribed, as a temporary measure, to promote evacuation while the patient tries to reestablish a normal bowel routine. The laxative may then be gradually withdrawn.

CU's medical consultants suggest that you avoid laxatives containing ingredients that act as bowel stimulants, unless advised by your physician. These drugs include phenolphthalein

(*Ex-Lax, Feen-A-Mint*), senna (*Fletcher's Castoria, Laxaid, Senokot*), bisacodyl (*Dulcolax*), and cascara (*Cas-Evac*). All these agents stimulate peristalsis and are capable of producing severe painful cramping.

A second class of laxatives, which also produces its effects by increasing peristalsis, includes saline (salt) cathartics. The most popular salts used are magnesium hydroxide (milk of magnesia) and sodium phosphate (*Phospho-Soda, Sal Hepatica*). Results with these laxatives can be dramatic, depending on the dose used. Patients with chronic kidney disease, who may have difficulty in excreting magnesium, should be wary about using milk of magnesia. And patients on salt-restricted diets should avoid laxatives containing sodium.

Consumers Union's medical consultants recommend that — if you must resort to a laxative — you restrict yourself to a bulk-producing laxative or a stool softener. Bulk-producing laxatives, such as pysillium (*Effersyllium, Mucilose, Plova, Syllamalt*) and methylcellulose (*Cellothyl*) tend to cause fewer unpleasant side effects than bowel irritants. Stool softeners work for some people, but not for all. These detergent products act to permit fluids to penetrate the stool, and thereby increase its water content. Dioctyl sodium sulfosuccinate is the main detergent or softener in clinical use, and is marketed under such brand names as *Colace, Coloctyl, Dio Medicone, Disonate*, and *Doxinate*.

Mineral oil has had many loyal fans, particularly among the geriatric age group. However, use of mineral oil over a period of time may lead to lipid pneumonia, a chronic condition caused by inhalation of oil into the lungs. Because of this and other disadvantages such as rectal leakage and interference with the body's absorption of vitamins A, D, and E, mineral oil is no longer a laxative of choice.

The brand names on the preceding pages by no means exhaust the list of laxatives marketed through pharmacies and supermarkets. In addition to the single-ingredient preparations identified above, there is a large contingent of combination-type laxatives. Shoppers may find products combining a stool softener with a bulk laxative, or a bowel irritant with an emollient. As always, consumers are urged to read the label carefully. CU's medical consultants advise buying a product with only one active ingredient.

Yogurt and acidophilus milk once had quite a vogue for the treatment of bowel disorders, including constipation. The nutritive value of yogurt and other fermented milks is essentially the same as that of the whole milk from which they are made, hence they are good foods. But, although fermented milks have occasionally been reported successful in the treatment of mild constipation, they usually are not of much value. Nor is there any evidence to support the routine use of vitamin B_1, B_6, or any other vitamin in the treatment of habitual constipation.

Constipation in children requires special consideration. In the great majority of cases it is due to oversolicitous attitudes on the part of parents. When a child senses anxiety in a parent about bowel function, the child too may become tense and be unable to relax, and relaxation is essential to a normal bowel movement.

If constipation develops in a child, what should be done? A good rule to follow in treating a child's constipation is "Don't." A child will not become ill from a temporary lapse, and in a day or two normal bowel activity usually reestablishes itself spontaneously. If constipation is due to an acute ailment, medical supervision and nursing care for the acute illness, not laxatives, are required. If constipation tends to recur, it may be due to improper diet or bowel habits, and a physician should be consulted. The prohibition of laxatives, suppositories, and enemas for most children with constipation cannot be too strongly urged.

Chapter 9

Hemorrhoids and other anal disorders

FEW AREAS OF THE BODY are associated with so many inhibitions, fears, and fixations as the rectum and the anus. The anus is the body opening through which solid waste matter (feces) passes from the rectum. It is composed of circular muscle fibers, and its many nerve endings render it a very sensitive area. The rectum is the portion of the lower bowel, just above the anus, that leads from the part of the large bowel known as the sigmoid colon. The anorectal area is susceptible to three major disorders — itching, bleeding, and pain — which, either singly or in combination, may eventually require medical advice.

Many people are reluctant to consult a physician about problems in the anorectal area — some because of shyness, others because of fear that cancer might be to blame. In fact, cancer and other tumors practically never occur in the anus. They do develop in the rectum, often without causing pain or bleeding in the early stages. Prior to causing symptoms, they can be detected only through routine, periodic rectal examination by a physician, either digitally, or preferably with a lighted tube called a sigmoidoscope.

Most disorders in the anorectal region are nonmalignant and, if given timely medical care, can be cured or relieved quickly. The most common of these disorders is hemorrhoids.

Hemorrhoids, also called piles, are clusters of dilated, or varicose, veins in the lower rectum or anus. They usually occur between the ages of thirty and fifty; it is likely that a third or more of the population suffers from them. Many people have both internal hemorrhoids, which may bleed but are usually painless, and the external type, which can be very painful indeed.

When the blood clots in one of these distended veins, a painful condition known as a thrombosed hemorrhoid results. The pain of a thrombosed hemorrhoid can be formidable, and is aggravated by sitting, walking, sneezing, or coughing. Relief from this acute condition usually takes place when the clot is released by means of spontaneous rupture of the vein or by a surgical incision. Warm sitz baths (see below) may also prove successful, but usually take several days to bring relief.

Perhaps the most important factor in the development of hemorrhoids is chronic constipation (see Chapter 8). Habitual forceful straining to move the bowels leads to congestion and stretching of the veins of the rectum and anus. Too frequent use of laxatives may cause explosive types of bowel movements, which over a period of time produce the same undesirable results.

In women hemorrhoids frequently occur during or after pregnancy, as a result of increased pressure in the anal and rectal veins. Many people have noticed that after alcoholic drinks the stools tend to be looser or the bowels tend to move more frequently than usual, and that such a change in bowel habits, even though temporary, may provoke an attack of piles. And people with occupations requiring constant sitting or standing, or lifting of heavy objects, tend to suffer from hemorrhoids. In others, thrombosed piles often show up right after exercise requiring unusual strain.

The pain of external hemorrhoids may be relieved considerably by warm sitz baths, three or four times daily, for fifteen minutes at a time. A warm bath eases pain by relaxing the spasm of the sphincter muscles around the anus. Lying down also helps by eliminating the pressure caused by gravity.

Suppositories, although widely advertised, are of little proven value for either internal or external hemorrhoids. The most popular ingredients of such suppositories are bismuth salts, topical anesthetics such as benzocaine, vasoconstrictors such as ephedrine, and antiseptics such as oxyquinoline or phenylmercuric nitrate. Although the vasoconstrictor drugs in a suppository may be capable of checking minor capillary bleeding, they cannot be relied upon to check bleeding from a varicose vein. The latter type of bleeding usually stops by itself in a day or two, as soon as the pressure within the vein is relieved. However, *all* cases of rectal bleeding — new, persistent, or recurrent even after a year's interval — merit consultation with a physician.

Nor do suppositories have any beneficial effect on the pain of hemorrhoids. When a suppository is inserted in the anus, it passes by the painful hemorrhoids and slips upward into or beyond the pain-insensitive rectum before melting. If one must use a suppository, it might make more sense to make it into a paste and apply it directly to the anal area. Indeed, such over-the-counter ointments or salves may be useful medications when applied directly to painful or bleeding areas.

Ointments containing such anesthetic drugs as benzocaine or Pontocaine seem to have a mild pain- or itch-relieving effect in some cases of external hemorrhoids. There is no convincing evidence that the highly advertised *Preparation H* — an ointment reported to contain a material derived from yeast cells, shark liver oil, and phenylmercuric nitrate — is any more effective in relieving pain than other ointments. According to *The Medical Letter*, "There is no acceptable evidence substantiating advertised claims that *Preparation H* can shrink hemorrhoids, reduce inflammation, and heal injured tissue."

External hemorrhoids will generally become symptom-free by themselves if bowel function is improved. Neither electrocoagulation nor chemical cauterization is considered good practice, because these methods do not cure and they may cause secondary hemorrhage. Injection treatment has been largely discarded and is no longer widely used.

Severe cases of hemorrhoids may require surgery. In most instances, surgery cures existing hemorrhoids permanently. But, because not all the rectal or anal veins can be removed, there is always a possibility that new hemorrhoids will develop.

There are several new nonsurgical techniques for dealing with hemorrhoids, but not all medical authorities agree as to their effectiveness. These methods include the tying off of hemorrhoidal veins with rubber bands, anal dilatation treatments, and a newer technique which involves quick freezing of the hemorrhoids with specially designed instruments. Wide publicity has been give these procedures, and each has its ardent supporters. However, CU's medical consultants believe that more studies are required before any of these new treatments can be accepted for routine medical use.

Hemorrhoids are not usually a cause of anal itching. Occasionally, a definable and possibly treatable skin disorder in or around the anal canal is responsible. In other cases, itching may be a symptom of a general disease, such as diabetes, or it may come from infestation of the intestines by pinworms or roundworms; these causes of itching are treatable. Many times, however, no specific cause can be established; emotions probably play a significant role in many cases of chronic anal itch.

A lack of knowledge of the specific cause of anal itching in most patients has led to the use of many treatments of doubtful value, including anesthetic ointments, alcohol injections, tattooing of the skin with mercury, X ray, and even more radical procedures, such as excision of the skin. But all these measures have now been largely supplanted by application of ointments and salves containing cortisone or one of its numerous derivatives. Although many patients need to use the medication indefinitely, in most cases those who use it find that they remain virtually free of symptoms.

This method is generally not effective in treating the anal itching caused by oral antibiotics — particularly such broad-spectrum antibiotics as tetracycline or ampicillin. Such an itch may develop not only during the course of antibiotic treatment, but as late as a week or two afterward. This type of anal itch may be very resistant to treatment of any kind, but it usually disappears spontaneously, although it may take a long time. The use of lactobacillus tablets or yogurt has not been shown to be effective in either prevention or treatment. Some physicians may administer an antifungal agent with the antibiotic, but convincing proof that this is effective is lacking.

Anal fissures, which are small tears in the skin surrounding the anus, may be a cause of both rectal pain and itching. Since these fissures are usually small and inconspicuous, diagnosis must almost always be made by a physician. Treatment of anal fissures generally consists in keeping the area clean by means of sitz baths. In the intervals between baths ordinary talcum powder must be used to keep the area dry.

Self-treatment of any of the various rectal or anal disorders with nonprescription ointments or suppositories not only may aggravate the trouble and sensitize the skin, but as a result serious conditions may be overlooked. The only safe course is to seek medical care as soon as symptoms appear.

Chapter 10

Acne

ALTHOUGH ACNE is not a fatal disease and only occasionally causes pain or disfiguring scars, it can be a severe test of the emotional stamina of adolescents and their families. It usually comes at a time in life when increasing maturity is striving for expression, and appearance has assumed enormous importance. In our society — especially among adolescents — a clean, smooth skin, free of blemishes, seems to be the symbol of beauty and social acceptance.

For hundreds of years there has been a persistent belief that acne is in some mysterious way associated with sexual wishes, fantasies, or masturbation. This is simply not true. Acne may also be considered by some thoughtless persons to be the stigmata of physical, mental, and social inferiority. This too is obviously false. Nevertheless, acne often causes immeasurable mental anguish to those afflicted. The advertisers of many skin preparations for teenagers play on such anxieties in promoting their products.

Parents can make a real contribution if they try to help their children understand the nature of acne and do not dismiss genuine concern as mere vanity. Armed with the information in this chapter, teenagers will be far less susceptible to the blandishments of misleading advertising.

To understand why some self-help measures can play a role in acne care but also why over-the-counter (OTC) medication is so problematical, one needs to know what body mechanisms lead to acne. *Acne* (eruption of the face) *vulgaris* (common) is primarily a disorder of the pilosebaceous units of certain parts of the body. Each pilosebaceous unit consists of a hair follicle — from which a hair shaft protrudes — and a sebaceous gland that secretes sebum (a whitish fatty substance) into the follicle and through the pores to the surface of the skin adjacent to the hair shaft. The normal follicle is lined with cells that age, die, and are easily extruded through the pores of the skin. In time, these cells are replaced by younger ones and the cycle is repeated. Recent studies at the University of Oregon have shown that in acne patients the wall of the hair follicle is abnormal, and the older dead cells accumulate in layers, thus giving rise to the plugging of pores that is characteristic of acne.

The primary lesions of acne are comedones (whiteheads) — collections of cells, sebum, and bacteria that plug the shaft of the hair follicle. (Comedones that are exposed to the air become blackheads.) The secondary lesions of acne include papules, which occur when the pilosebaceous units become inflamed and protrude above the surface of the skin; pustules, which occur when the papules become pus-filled; and acne cysts, which are also inflammatory lesions but both larger and more deeply embedded in the skin than papules or pustules. Pimple — a popular term not used by dermatologists — is the common designation for a papule or pustule. To describe a patient's acne a physician may use the terms mild, moderate, or severe.

The inflammatory lesions of acne (papules, pustules, and cysts) result from the disruption of the follicle wall due to the presence of irritant substances within the follicle. Free fatty acids in sebum are thought to be the major irritants responsible for this disruption of the follicle wall and subsequent release of sebum into the skin around the follicle. CU's medical consultants report that there is considerable investigation under way to determine the origin of these fatty acids. Current research points to resident bacteria within the follicle as the culprit. These bacteria produce lipases — enzymes that break down the sebum into the irritant free fatty acids.

There are wide variations in the amount of sebum secreted in different areas of the skin. The most active sebaceous glands are located in the scalp, followed in descending order of activity by the forehead, face, chest, and upper back. Except for the scalp, areas with the highest sebum content are the most frequent sites of acne.

As part of the natural growth process, the sebaceous glands at puberty increase in size and secrete more sebum under the influence of increasing amounts of sex hormones, principally the male hormone. The increase in sebum production, combined with obstruction of the pores, sets the stage for the development of acne. If the overactivity of the sebaceous glands or the plugging of the pores could be better controlled, acne might pose less of a problem.

Animal experiments have shown that the sex hormones — testosterone, progesterone, and estrogen — affect sebaceous activity. Testosterone and progesterone stimulate the sebaceous glands, while estrogen tends to reduce their activity. Estrogen, however, must be taken in fairly large doses — so large, in fact, as to produce undesirable side effects in the male — if it is to reduce sebaceous gland secretion to a degree that may be significant in acne. Consequently, the use of estrogen has been — and should be — reserved for females with severe cases of acne. Such therapy, however, may be inadvisable in a still-growing female because it may stunt growth. When estrogen is prescribed for acne in a female who has attained full growth, it is often given in combination with a progestin (as in an oral contraceptive) in order to prevent irregular menstrual flow.

Unless acne is severe, however, a visit to the doctor is not usually necessary. According to a CU medical consultant, only one acne patient in ten requires medical attention. Most mild or moderate cases respond to effective OTC medication (see table on page 119) and to home care.

A wide variety of OTC acne products is available. Besides the creams, cleansers, lotions, soaps, powders, and gels one might expect, drugstores sell cleansing sticks, a variety of scrubs, impregnated towelettes, tablets, and many other items. Except for cosmetic agents designed solely to hide the lesions and to blend with the surrounding skin, many of these products contain the same more or less time-honored medicaments that have been tried by physicians over the years in the management of this stubborn ailment.

Ingredients commonly used in OTC remedies and believed by most dermatologists to be of some value are benzoyl peroxide, sulfur, resorcinol, and salicylic acid (see table on page 119). All four inflame the skin and cause it to peel. Benzoyl peroxide is the strongest, creating the most inflammation and peeling — and often the most improvement. It occurs in adequate concentrations in several OTC products (such as *Benoxyl, Loroxide, Oxy-5, Persadox,* and *Vanoxide*). Milder preparations that may be effective are those containing at least 2 percent sulfur. Less likely to be effective are those products with less than 2 percent sulfur or those depending just on resorcinol. Remedies with less than 2 percent resorcinol or salicylic acid as their only effective agent are probably too weak to do any good.

Because each person's skin differs in sensitivity and each person's acne problem differs in magnitude, no single acne product is ideal for everyone. If your skin is sensitive and your acne mild, try a formulation that is not as strong as benzoyl peroxide — a sulfur/resorcinol or sulfur/salicylic acid combination. If your skin is of tougher fiber and your acne moderate, start with a benzoyl peroxide formulation. If the product seems unsuitable — too weak or too harsh — switch accordingly. It is important to follow directions carefully. These agents are capable of causing injury if used in too high a concentration or too often without medical supervision. If your skin becomes overly dry and scaly — even with a mild product — stop applications for a while and also cut down on your use of soap. If discomfort or scaliness persists, consult a physician.

Avoid products that do not include any of the four effective ingredients on their labels. Some preparations may list one or more of the four effective ingredients, but the labels do not always specify percentages. Such an omission may often signify inadequate amounts of active ingredients. Accordingly, CU's medical consultants suggest that you also avoid a product if the label does not state the percentage of each ingredient.

Distrust the claims of an acne product's label or packaging. "An aid in the relief of acne pimples and blackheads," is printed on the label of *PropaPh*, even though the product contains no ingredients known to improve acne. *Noxzema Skin Cream* claims to "help heal those blemishes for a clean, clear look." But it, too, contains none of the four ingredients most dermatologists agree are effective.

How informative are the ads? Not very. *Tackle*, "the stinger working on those blemishes" — the supposedly "strong medication" — contains 2 percent of resorcinol as its only effective antiacne agent. The medicine in *Stri-Dex Medicated Pads* "can get into your pores and kill bacteria that can cause skin infection." Maybe, but not deep enough to kill the bacteria that contribute to acne. *Clearasil* is "the most serious kind of blemish medicine you can get without a prescription," according to a television commercial. *Clearasil* does contain a potent sulfur/resorcinol combination, but so do several other OTC antiacne aids. In November 1973 the Federal Trade Commission ordered fourteen manufacturers of acne preparations (including *PropaPH*, *Noxzema*, and *Clearasil*) to substantiate advertising slogans.

Acne patients whose skin has not responded to OTC medication may wish to consult a physician. And certainly all those with severe cases of acne should seek medical help to prevent destruction of tissue and to minimize the possibility of permanent scarring. CU's medical consultants suggest, if you need medical help for your acne, that you first consult your family physician. Your doctor can then decide whether to take on your case or to refer you to a dermatologist. No physician can cure acne — only time can do that. But a doctor can prescribe medication specifically tailored to each patient's needs with dosage and proportion of ingredients adjusted individually.

Antibiotics, in usual therapeutic dosages, have been prescribed by physicians to treat particularly severe cases of acne. In recent years, doctors have noticed that smaller doses of broad-spectrum antibiotics, administered daily for long periods of time (months or even years), have had a beneficial effect on many acne patients. This low-dose antibiotic therapy has been shown to reduce the concentration of inflammation-producing free fatty acids. Acne researchers believe that antibiotics cause a decline in the amount of free fatty acid by decreasing the number of bacteria in the follicle, thereby limiting the amount of bacterial lipases present. Many patients can safely continue low-dose antibiotic therapy under medical supervision for months or even years. Side effects from such use are generally minimal, barring allergic reactions.

Antibiotics are sometimes put in OTC creams or ointments; there is no evidence that such products will prevent, relieve, or cure acne. Indeed, they may compound the problem by causing an allergic reaction when applied to the skin.

The most recent addition to acne therapy is vitamin A acid (retinoic acid), which was cleared by the Food and Drug Administration (FDA) in 1972 as a topical preparation for prescription use only. In a controlled study, retinoic acid was found superior to benzoyl peroxide and to a sulfur/resorcinol lotion in producing irritation and peeling. However, patience is required; the acne may even appear to worsen during the first six weeks of treatment. Improvement is rarely seen before three to four months.

In addition to the usual irritative changes, an occasional patient may also experience a photosensitivity reaction (an intense reaction to sunlight resulting in skin reddening and painful blistering — see page 155) as well as mild loss of skin pigment. According to *The Medical Letter*, some clinicians believe that vitamin A acid therapy "represents an advance" in the treatment of acne, although there is no conclusive evidence yet "that this drug is superior to traditional chemical peeling agents. . . "

In addition to the new topical use of vitamin A acid, the taking of vitamin A in large doses by mouth has long had its advocates. In true vitamin A deficiency, the skin and the mucous membrane, including the lining of the hair follicle, become thickened and horny. Since in acne similar changes occur in the hair follicle, some doctors have reasoned that extralarge doses of vitamin A may prevent or cure acne. In most cases, however, the treatment has been unsuccessful. In one fairly large study, a group of college students with acne were given 100,000 units of vitamin A a day — about twenty times the recommended daily allowance. Slightly more than half of them showed some improvement — but so did half of a control group that received only a placebo. Taking vitamin A in doses greater than 50,000 units a day for several months has been followed in some people by loss of body hair, skin itching, enlargement of the liver and spleen, and a feeling of pressure inside the head. Such treatment is advocated by some authorities for short-term therapy in severe cases but needs close professional supervision. The FDA has required since October 1973 that vitamin A in a dosage larger than 10,000 international units be bought only on prescription and not be treated as an OTC drug.

The antiacne arsenal available to doctors also includes the injection of corticosteroids into acne cysts, cryotherapy (freeze technique), and incision and drainage of infected cysts. However, none of these treatments is yet capable of eliminating acne. A promising area of current research centers on drugs that reduce sebum formation without the side effects of estrogen. Some scientists foresee a major breakthrough when they learn more about the disruption of the follicle wall (see page 110).

In treatment of acne, dermatologists recommend that the face be washed several times daily with soap and warm water. There is no actual proof that facewashing helps. However, scrubbing with a soapy washcloth does remove some oils, dead skin, and surface bacteria. It also produces minor irritation, which may be of some help in mild acne.

In any case, CU's medical consultants do not believe that success in treatment depends on the type of soap used. Ordinary soap usually does an adequate job cleansing the skin. Such heavily advertised cleansing products as *Noxzema Skin Cream*, *PHisoDerm Medicated Liquid*, and *Cuticura Medicated Soap* are no more useful than a bar of plain soap. "Acne soaps" with sulfur are not particularly helpful because the medication is likely to wash away. Although some doctors may prefer tincture of green soap to ordinary soap, CU's medical consultants do not consider it of any special value.

Disregard the word "antibacterial" on the label of acne products. While antibacterial soaps are indeed effective in reducing the number of skin bacteria, there are hazards in using these products (see page 155). Moreover, antibacterial soaps — which may be of some usefulness in certain areas (the armpits, for example) — are not at all relevant for acne therapy. Although bacteria are the source of the enzymes that break down oils into irritating free fatty acids, these bacteria live beneath the skin's surface, deep in the follicles. They cannot be reached by hexachlorophene (now available only by prescription) or by its antibacterial successors in cleansing products. Advertising claims to the contrary are without basis.

Of some value for certain people are abrasive soaps, such as *Brasivol* and *Pernox*, which contain irritating granules. These products physically induce the therapeutic inflammation and peeling that antiacne medications cause chemically. But they can be quite harsh to sensitive skin. Those who want to experiment should start by using an abrasive soap once a day. If the skin tolerates it, it can be used more frequently; if not, it should be used only occasionally or not at all.

Many women, influenced by cosmetic advertising, have developed the habit of using face creams in place of soap and water for cleansing the face. This is of dubious value for those with acne, because greases and creams encourage plugging of the pores. All so-called skin foods, skin tonics, lubricating creams, and vanishing creams should be avoided, too.

Even though the desire to cover up blemishes may be overwhelming, it's best not to use any cosmetics. For those who feel they must use cosmetics, water-based products, applied lightly, are the least likely to cause complications. If the hair is naturally oily, it should be kept off the face. Although acne lesions do not occur in the scalp, avoid hair dressings with greasy or lanolin bases. Long-term use of such preparations can cause "pomade acne," a clustering of blackheads on the forehead and temples. Correction of dandruff seems to be beneficial in some cases of acne. Shampoo at least once, preferably twice, a week; frequent washing does not damage hair or scalp (see Chapter 11).

Ultraviolet (UV) rays from sunlight or a sunlamp are helpful in acne when they cause a reddening and slight scaling of the skin, but the danger of overexposure resulting in severe facial burns often outweighs any benefits. The eyelids are particularly vulnerable to UV radiation (see Chapter 14).

One of the prime temptations with acne is to pick and squeeze at blackheads and plump pimples. Resist it. Handling acne blemishes can spread infections, rupture follicle walls, and may lead eventually to deep-pitted scars. If you feel compelled to remove blackheads, buy a blackhead extractor from a pharmacy. Before you use it, soften the plugged pores by applying warm water compresses for a few minutes.

Since products containing iodides or bromides sometimes exacerbate existing acne or produce eruptions that look like acne, patients are warned against them during acne treatment. Certain drugs, such as cough medicines, sedatives, cold medications, and multivitamin/mineral combinations, may contain iodides or bromides. (Bromides have now been eliminated from some OTC preparations, such as *Bromo Seltzer*.) Since iodides also occur in iodized salt, saltwater fish, shellfish, spinach, cabbage, lettuce, and artichokes, these foods should be avoided.

Most authorities agree that any other type of dietary manipulation usually makes no difference in the severity of acne vulgaris; at least one double-blind study supports such a hypothesis. With some people, however, it may seem that specific foods do aggravate the disease. The foods usually implicated in acne are sweets, nuts, chocolate, and fried foods. If it seems that any food worsens the acne, try dropping it from your diet and observe the effect (if any). After a few weeks, reintroduce the food and again note the result. If the experiment convinces you that the food is suspect, try to avoid it completely. More likely you will find that changes in your diet make little difference and that you can eat what you like.

If careful trial of OTC medications (see table on page 119), skin cleansing, and possibly elimination of certain foodstuffs do not help, a physician should be consulted both to verify the diagnosis and as a guide to treatment. Control of acne may not come with the first round of treatment. Those who consult a doctor for acne should be encouraged to be patient in follow-

OTC acne products

CU's medical consultants urge you to read the label before you buy an acne preparation. The four OTC antiacne ingredients likely to be effective in the treatment of mild or moderate cases are benzoyl peroxide, sulfur, resorcinol, and salicylic acid. Product labels, however, do not always list the amount of each ingredient. CU's medical consultants have prepared the following guide to some OTC acne preparations on the market. Listings of these products are based on the presence of an effective ingredient in an adequate amount (see page 112).

PRODUCTS LIKELY TO BE HELPFUL

Acnaveen	*Clearasil*	*PHisoAc*
Acne	*Contrablem*	*Resulin*
Acne Aid	*Fostex*	*Rezamid*
Acnomel	*Fostril*	*Sulforcin*
Acnycin	*Klaron*	*Thera-Blem*
Benoxyl	*Loroxide*	*Transact*
Bensulfoid	*Oxy-5*	*Vanoxide*
Cenac	*Persadox*	

PRODUCTS LESS LIKELY TO BE HELPFUL

Medicated Face Conditioner	*Teenac*
Queen Helene Mint Julep Masque	*Ten-O-Six*
Stri-Dex Medicated Pads	*Therapads*
Tackle	*Therapads Plus*

PRODUCTS NOT LIKELY TO BE HELPFUL

Cuticura Medicated Soap	*Pro-Blem*
Ice-O-Derm	*PropaPH*
Jergens Clear Complexion Gel	*Revlon Natural Wonder Super Clean-up*
Noxzema Skin Cream	*Sebacide*
PHisoDerm Medicated Liquid	*Seba-Nil*

ing subsequent directions. It may help if you keep in mind that acne, which responds slowly to a physician's care, is likely to be even more stubborn with hit-or-miss self-medication.

While found predominantly in teenagers, acne is not at all uncommon in young adults, particularly women. Dermatologists who treat "adult acne" have found more often than not that patients in their twenties with adult acne did not have acne as teenagers. The abrupt onset of acne in middle age may be a symptom of an endocrine disorder, and merits consultation with a physician.

Chapter 11

Dandruff and shampoos

WHATEVER THEIR ADVOCATES say about new dandruff "cures" and medicinal shampoos, there has been no real progress in the prevention or treatment of dandruff in recent years. Advertising campaigns have kept the public acutely aware of dandruff, and have promoted scores of remedies for actual and fancied scalp disorders. In a few cases claims have been so wild and so obviously false that the Federal Trade Commission has stepped in with cease-and-desist orders.

Oiliness and flakiness of the scalp are normal. The human scalp, even at its healthiest, shows a mild degree of scaling; the skin all over the body continually sloughs off bits of its dead outer layer. On the scalp, sebaceous glands add their oily secretion (sebum) to the dead skin scales. This combination forms dandruff.

Most dandruff is nothing more than this normal phenomenon, and a reasonably clean and healthy scalp can be maintained by shampooing once or twice a week with shampoo (or soap, in a soft water area). If there is much dirt in the air, or if there is excessive sweating, shampooing more frequently is in order. Even daily shampooing, if it seems needed, does not harm the hair or scalp. Brushing may serve to tidy the hair, but does not alleviate dandruff. In fact, some authorities believe

121

that excessive brushing may even damage the hair, especially if the brush has nylon or other synthetic bristles.

The main purpose in shampooing is to cleanse the hair of sebum, dead skin scales, and ordinary dirt. Obviously, it is better if the shampoo can function without removing all the natural oils. CU's medical consultants prefer soap shampoos, which are hard to find. Soap shampoos may be slightly more protective of the hair cuticle (outer coat) but may not cleanse as well as detergent brands, especially in hard water. To compensate for any possible harshness, various additives are used in detergent shampoos — for example, lanolin, which is purported to replace natural oils. Other additives are put in shampoos to meet special needs. For instance, people who think their hair could use more "body" may wish to use shampoos with protein conditioners which coat the hair to give it a thicker appearance. (Despite claims for some brands, any systemic benefits from these protein products have not been proved.) Cream rinses may help neutralize the negative electric charge in newly shampooed hair, thus preventing "fly-away" hair and making the hair easier to comb.

But dandruff control is not always that simple. Sometimes the production of oily secretions and dead skin scales speeds up until the flaking is definitely excessive. Transition from the normal to the abnormal state is so gradual that it is difficult to tell when one condition ends and the other begins.

Severe dandruff, which is not uncommon, may require treatment by a physician. Its precise cause is unknown. There is no basis for assuming, as some advertisers do, that germs are the primary cause and that an antiseptic shampoo is the cure. Indeed, although severe dandruff can be controlled, it cannot be completely cured. Spontaneous improvement is common, irrespective of the kind of treatment applied, a fact that casts doubt on all testimonials for cures with any particular product.

Dandruff is often confused with another scalp condition, seborrhea, in which there is an excessive amount of sebum. In the scalp this condition is characterized by very oily hair. It is common during the teenage years when the sebaceous glands are extremely active (see Chapter 10). Sometimes redness and itching are associated with seborrhea; the forehead, nose, cheeks, and even the upper chest are occasionally involved. It is then called seborrheic dermatitis and requires a physician's attention. Shampoos effective against seborrheic dermatitis can be obtained on prescription.

The classic and still effective drugs that doctors use to treat seborrheic dermatitis may include sulfur, selenium sulfide, salicylic acid, zinc pyrithione, and tar. Such ingredients are fairly effective and usually safe. A prescription may call for one of these drugs alone, or for a combination mixed together in various proportions in ointments or lotions. The kind of ointment or lotion and the concentration and choice of ingredients depend on the severity of the condition. The medication may be prescribed to be rubbed in at night and washed out in the morning with an ordinary shampoo.

Some over-the-counter (OTC) remedies make use of one or more of the classic drugs, usually with the addition of other less rational ingredients, but such ready-made products are at a disadvantage. The proportions of ingredients cannot be tailored to the patient; and when the product is self-administered, there is no trained eye to evaluate the effectiveness and adjust matters accordingly. In general, all claims made for OTC dandruff remedies should be viewed with a skeptical eye.

There is no evidence that changes in diet or the addition of vitamins or minerals to the diet can control the development of dandruff or affect the quality of the hair in the slightest way. Nor is there any evidence that exposure of the scalp or head to sunlight either prevents or cures any type of scalp disorder.

Many men worry that dandruff might lead to baldness. Although severe dandruff and the male type of baldness (begin-

ning at the temples and progressing to form a "widow's peak")
may occur simultaneously, no cause-and-effect relationship
between them has ever been shown. There are also innumer-
able instances in which dandruff and scalp oiliness last for years
without leading to the slightest thinning of the hair. It should
be remembered that it is normal to lose a certain number of
hairs daily. And normally they are replaced by newly grown
hairs.

In the male, male-type baldness generally appears in early
adult life without being preceded or accompanied by any
marked oiliness or dandruff. This type of baldness is inherited.
It and other types of baldness are not cured by local remedies
or by manipulation of the scalp; nor are drugs, hormones, or
any other agents taken by mouth of use. Some men have re-
sorted to hair transplants, but the procedure requires an experienced professional. Male-type baldness in a female may be the
result of an endocrine disorder.

Chapter 12

First aid
for wounds,
burns, and bites

NORMAL SKIN IS A RUGGED ORGAN built to withstand considerable assault. Its mild acidity, oily coating, and horny outer layer of dead cells can protect the underlying living skin quite well. The skin's outer layer is subject to the constant erosive effect of day-to-day living, including bathing, scratching, rubbing, and other conscious and unconscious activities. These outer cells are continuously sloughed off, to be replaced in an orderly fashion by other younger cells from the subepidermal layers. Thus the skin is a constantly self-renewing organ, ever changing, and not the static structure many people assume it to be.

So long as the outer layer is intact, most of the things — medicinal or otherwise — that reach the skin either intentionally or by accident cannot do much damage. When this barrier is breached, however, as it is when there is a cut, scratch, rash, or other irritation, any topical preparation can penetrate more easily, with possibly damaging results.

Left alone, injured or inflamed skin has remarkable recuperative powers. Treated with the wrong chemical, it may find the double assault just too much and medication dermatitis may result. The skin may react with itching, redness, burning, rash, blisters, or even a crusted, oozing dermatitis. In some instances, additional self-treatment has led to reactions severe enough to result in hospitalization. The truth is that most skin ailments are better off without the many topical remedies found among the thousands of over-the-counter (OTC) preparations currently on the market.

SCRATCHES, CUTS, AND ABRASIONS

Scratches, cuts, and other small wounds can best be treated by cleansing with soap, thoroughly rinsing under running tap water, and covering with a small bandage for protection from additional contamination. Those who feel they must use an antiseptic should shun the highly promoted brand-name products, choosing instead isopropyl (rubbing) alcohol. Like most antiseptics, alcohol should be applied, if at all, on the intact skin around the wound, not in the wound.

The makers of branded antiseptic products do not share these views; indeed, in their advertising they often imply dire consequences if their products are not used. But whatever the advertisements and labels say, the truth is that first-aid antiseptic salves, sprays, and solutions probably do no good, and may at times actually retard healing. The impact of these products varies to some extent with the type and amount of active ingredients in each preparation's formula. The agents most commonly used in first-aid antiseptic products fall into several categories:

ALCOHOLS. Most frequently isopropyl or ethyl alcohol is used. The former is much cheaper and just as effective. Isopropyl (70 percent) alcohol, usually purchased as rubbing alcohol, is probably as effective in killing most skin bacteria as any other type of germicide in common use. For first-aid use, alcohol is considered the most effective and least irritating of all antiseptics and is virtually devoid of allergic effects.

Tinctures (alcoholic solutions) are generally more effective than aqueous (water) solutions of a given germicide. But alcohol alone is as effective as an equal amount of many tinctures.

ANTIBIOTICS. Antibiotic preparations intended for use on the skin are available without a doctor's prescription. Neomycin and bacitracin are the antibiotics most commonly used. The wisdom of using antibiotics without medical supervision is to be questioned (see Chapter 28). The use of antibiotics can lead to infections by resistant microorganisms, and allergic reactions are frequently reported.

BISPHENOLS (bithionol, hexachlorophene). Bisphenols, if used consistently, are effective in reducing the number of bacteria on the skin surface, but they do not kill the bacteria as quickly or as completely as alcohol. In 1972 the Food and Drug Administration banned the use of hexachlorophene in OTC products in concentrations strong enough to be effective as an antiseptic. Products that formerly relied on it — such as *Medi-Quik* and *Solarcaine* — have been reformulated using other antibacterials.

HALOGENS (principally iodine). These antiseptics are most often available as tinctures. Aqueous solutions of iodine compounds (*Betadine, Isodine*) have also been marketed. They cause less staining of the skin and less stinging, and are almost as effective as tinctures for first-aid use; but they are more expensive. The iodine in these preparations can be absorbed even through intact skin. This can increase the blood iodide content which, although not harmful with occasional use, can interfere with certain thyroid function tests.

HEAVY-METAL COMPOUNDS. These include mercurial compounds (such as ammoniated mercury, phenylmercuric compounds, *Mercurochrome, Merthiolate, Metaphen*). Many are available both as tinctures and in aqueous solution. It has been shown that these compounds do not consistently kill bacteria with which they come in contact, although they may prevent these bacteria from actively multiplying. Allergic skin reactions are fairly common.

PHENOLS (carbolic acid, cresol). To be effective, phenol and phenol derivatives must be used in such high concentrations that they irritate the skin. Phenol itself is thought to penetrate the skin; if it does penetrate in sufficient quantity, systemic reactions, such as muscle tremors and convulsions, may occur. This chemical still shows up in some OTC remedies. And several brand-name antiseptic products, including *Listerine Antiseptic* and *S.T. 37 Antiseptic*, contain phenol derivatives.

QUATERNARY AMMONIUM COMPOUNDS (chiefly, benzalkonium chloride). These substances are effective against the two broad classes of bacteria (see page 295) — Gram-positive organisms, including staphylococci, commonly the cause of skin infections, and Gram-negative bacteria, which also cause skin infections. The latter, however, tend to be more resistant and require longer exposure to the antiseptic. OTC products containing this class of antiseptic include *Bactine*, *Phemerol Chloride*, and *Zephiran Chloride*.

Another product often found in home medicine cabinets is hydrogen peroxide in the usual 3 percent solution. Although it is a poor antiseptic, its frothing action may sometimes help to cleanse particularly dirty wounds.

CU's medical consultants do not recommend any antiseptic packaged as an aerosol spray. Not only are aerosols more expensive than bottled antiseptics, but their use may involve additional hazards (see page 311).

"First-aid creams" are actively promoted as aids in healing wounds, but this should not be taken to mean that they *speed* healing. Very few data are available to show how effective they actually are.

The widespread belief that every break in the skin should be treated with an antiseptic results mainly from needless anxiety about the large numbers of bacteria normally present on the skin surface at all times. Most of these bacteria are harmless. Indeed, one school of thought maintains that such microorganisms aid in maintaining a healthy skin. The majority of organisms that enter a wound are handled most effectively not by an applied germicide but by the body's natural defenses.

These defenses, which are not fully understood, nearly always seem able to cope with the bacteria in a small wound. Certainly, one of the defenses is the physical barrier offered by the skin itself. At the site of a wound, the body must rely on white blood cells and serum factors, which become concentrated in that area. These defenses are most effective when the skin is damaged as little as possible, and when conditions in and around the wound are as unfavorable to bacterial growth as possible.

With this background, it is not difficult to outline a rational program for the treatment of minor wounds — comparatively small scratches, cuts, or abrasions. Three steps are involved: cleansing the wound gently, cleansing the skin around the wound thoroughly, and protecting the wound from further contamination.

The cleansing of the wound itself should be gentle to avoid further injury, but foreign bodies — such as dirt or gravel — must be removed. Dead tissue and foreign matter in the wound provide an excellent medium for bacterial growth. Gentle scrubbing with a mild soap and water, followed by flushing with tap water, usually does a good job of cleansing the wound itself. Bits of foreign matter not removed this way should be lifted out as carefully as possible with tweezer tips wiped with alcohol. Spontaneous bleeding also helps to flush the wound and may be advantageous, particularly for superficial puncture wounds.

Most of the organisms that still remain after the washing can be eliminated by swabbing the skin around the wound with an antiseptic, preferably isopropyl (70 percent) alcohol. Within a few days a scab forms. It is not as effective a physical barrier as intact skin, but it helps protect the wound during healing.

If the wound becomes infected, yellowish pus will appear on the surface of the wound or under the scab. In that case, sterile, warm, wet compresses should be applied several times daily. Healing commences as the pus disappears.

Because a scab is easily broken, some additional protection is often advisable. A covering of sterile, unmedicated gauze and adhesive tape ordinarily suffices. The bandage should not be airtight, since it might then trap moisture given off by the skin and encourage the growth of bacteria. Plastic adhesive tape, unless it is "breathable," is unsatisfactory in this respect. If the wound is more of a scrape than a cut, one of the plastic "non-stickable" coverings may be helpful because they usually do not stick to the wound.

Small (less than 1-inch) lacerations will heal faster and with less scarring if the wound edges are brought together by two or three bridging pieces of tape. These are commonly known as "butterfly" bandages and can be made or purchased.

If the wound bleeds after a bandage is applied, and the bandage becomes stuck, it is best to leave it on as long as the wound is healing normally. Pulling the scab loose to change the dressing can only retard healing and increase the chances of infection. If a bandage must be removed, soaking it in warm water or hydrogen peroxide can help soften the scab and make removal easier.

Do not try self-medication or home treatment of any kind if you have a deep puncture wound (because of the difficulty in cleansing it through the small break in the skin) or a large cut or a badly lacerated wound (because of the danger of bacterial infection combined with the larger healing task confronting the body). Such wounds should be protected with a sterile dressing, and the patient should be taken promptly to a physician. Excessive bleeding from such wounds can usually be controlled by applying *firm* hand pressure over the wound (preferably using a clean cloth). *The use of a tourniquet is rarely if ever necessary* and may result in irreversible changes in an affected limb.

One possible complication from any wound is tetanus (commonly known as lockjaw). People can best avoid this often fatal disease by being immunized against the bacterium that causes it. CU's medical consultants join with the U.S. Public Health Service (PHS) in urging that everyone who has not been immunized against tetanus take the full series of three injections of tetanus toxoid (the first two a month apart, and the third seven months after the second). After this initial immunization — often completed in childhood — a booster injection is normally required only every ten years.

Even though an injured person has been fully immunized, a physician may decide that an additional booster is required. When past immunization appears inadequate, tetanus antitoxin (derived from *human*, not horse, serum) is usually administered along with the first injection of the three-part immunization schedule. Of course, the remaining two injections of tetanus toxoid should still be taken in the usual sequence.

BURNS

Burns, one of the most common of skin wounds, call for special consideration. They are classified according to the depth of damage. In a first-degree burn, there is reddening of the skin, caused by the dilatation of small blood vessels. In a second-degree burn, serum or fluid escapes from these vessels into the outer layer of the skin, causing blisters. In a third-degree burn, the entire depth of the skin and some subcutaneous tissues are destroyed. Only first-degree and small second-degree burns can be safely treated at home.

The pain of such burns can be relieved by immediate immersion of the affected part (for five to ten minutes or longer) in ice water or cold running water. Cold, wet compresses may also be useful as long as there is pain. This treatment not only soothes the pain but may also prevent blistering. A dressing, firmly applied, may also help to prevent blistering. If blistering does occur, the dressing will guard against rupture of the blisters, as well as secondary infection.

There is no evidence that butter, lard, or cooking grease of any kind — if applied to the burn — is of any value at all. Vitamin E ointment has been promoted by some manufacturers as useful for treating superficial burns; CU's medical consultants know of no controlled studies to support the claim.

Authorities on first aid and the treatment of burns recommend that OTC burn ointments never be used. Most of these remedies contain one or more of the following: an anesthetic (usually lidocaine or benzocaine), an antiseptic, menthol, lanolin, cod-liver oil, and vitamins. None of these materials has been shown to have any special pain-relieving value beyond that provided by the petroleum jelly or similar vehicle in which it is contained. Nor has it been established that OTC burn ointments are of value in preventing infection or in assisting healing; in some instances, ointments may even interefere with healing. Futhermore, the anesthetic and antiseptic ingredients in many commercial burn ointments have been known to cause allergic reactions.

Extensive burns (those involving more than just one or two areas of the body), irrespective of their depth, should be considered emergencies and treated by a physician as soon as possible. It is hazardous to apply any ointment, oil, salve, or solution to a third-degree burn, because the drugs in the preparation can be more readily absorbed and cause toxic reactions. The depth of the burn allows ready absorption of any applied medication, for there is no protective skin barrier. Also, OTC burn preparations can seriously interfere with later professional care.

Sunburn resembles an ordinary burn. If it is mild and without blistering, the pain may be relieved by compresses of cold water or by cool baths. Aspirin or acetaminophen in usual doses can help as well. Extensive sunburn or deep, blistered sunburn calls for medical treatment. (To prevent sunburn, see Chapter 14.)

BITES

Those who continually scratch mosquito bites only aggravate the symptoms and may risk infection. Itching, which may be severe, can be eased by applications of very cold or very hot compresses.

Insect repellents can be effective against many insects. In 1970 CU reviewed twenty-two brands of personal insect repellents and judged most effective those products using diethyl toluamide in the greatest concentration. Such products were found more likely to give longer-lasting protection against certain species of insects (not including spiders, wasps, or bees), to feel a little less oily, and to be harder to rub off or wash off than brands based on ethyl hexanediol.

Bites from insects in the class Hymenoptera (bees, wasps, hornets) can be a more serious matter. A nonallergic individual may experience various reactions, ranging from mild irritation and itching at the bite site to swelling of an entire extremity. Immediate treatment consists of removal of the stinger (should it remain), and application of very cold compresses. Anyone with serious symptoms from such a bite should see a physician. A few people are highly sensitive to the venom released by these insects. Even those who are subject to anaphylactic reactions (see page 298) — which can prove fatal — can be made relatively immune with appropriate injections by an allergist. Obviously, such people must still maintain continued caution and take protective measures against insect stings.

Bites by animals — domestic or wild — occur with some frequency, and because of the threat of rabies even a minor bite must receive careful attention. Although human rabies is rare in the United States, the Center for Disease Control reports that antirabies treatment is administered to about 30,000 people a year. Dogs and cats account for the majority of bites, but the most important sources of actual infection are wild animals such as skunks, foxes, coyotes, raccoons, and bats.

If a domestic pet just nicks you, the bite should be handled much as any slight wound is, as described earlier in this chapter. Even though bacterial infection is the main hazard of such a bite, careful cleansing of the wound in a routine manner can probably also decrease the chances of rabies transmission. In addition, adequate immunization against tetanus is necessary, and the advice of a physician may be required.

Even a slight scratch from a *wild* animal, which cannot be held for observation (see below), must be considered potentially rabid until proved otherwise, according to the PHS. In such instances, antirabies treatment should be initiated immediately.

For a more extensive bite from either a domestic or a wild animal, a visit to a physician becomes mandatory. (The PHS reports that rabies treatment is rarely needed for bites of rabbits, squirrels, chipmunks, rats, or mice.) An animal that has bitten a human being must be kept under observation for at least ten days. If it is rabid, it will die at some point within that period, and its brain can easily be examined for evidence of rabies. Should such examination be positive, a course of treatment with duck embryo rabies vaccine must be initiated at once. If the animal cannot be located, the physician will usually take into consideration the extent and location of the wound before recommending whether rabies vaccine should be administered. If the animal under observation remains well, no treatment for rabies is indicated.

Chapter 13

Treating poison ivy

POISON IVY DERMATITIS — the rash that follows contact with poison ivy, poison oak, or poison sumac — is one of the most common of all allergic disorders. And for its treatment numerous kinds of over-the-counter (OTC) preparations have been introduced over the years; unfortunately, there is no convincing evidence that any of these products is more effective than a few simple standard measures.

Although poison ivy dermatitis can be acquired in any season, the peak incidence occurs in springtime. The poisonous sap may reach susceptible skin not only through direct contact with the plant (or with its smoke if burned), but by way of shoes, clothing, tools, and the fur of domestic animals. Such intermediaries, however, may be made harmless by washing them with soap or a detergent. The common belief that the disease spreads as the blisters on the skin rupture is without scientific support.

Sensitivity to poison ivy varies markedly among different people, and even in different periods of a person's life. It is extremely unwise to assume that you have natural immunity to poison ivy, since apparent resistance one year may be followed by explosive sensitivity the next year. In general, the degree of sensitivity is highest in childhood and diminishes with age.

Farmers, foresters, and others who spend much time outdoors in areas where poison ivy plants are common often acquire a degree of resistance.

As a rule, poison ivy skin eruption appears one or two days after contact with the poisonous sap, and the eruption can be unpleasant indeed. Anyone who has had a serious case, or has seen someone with such a case, will not be surprised that many potions and treatments have been proposed to prevent or cure this allergic reaction. Among the many agents at one time thought to be beneficial in relieving poison ivy eruption were bromine, kerosene, gunpowder, iodine, buttermilk, cream, and marshmallows, as well as a large number of botanical preparations.

Strong laundry soap has long enjoyed popularity. However, Dr. Albert M. Kligman of the University of Pennsylvania Medical School, an authority on poison ivy dermatitis, has demonstrated that, in a highly sensitive person, washing delayed only five minutes after exposure does very little good; and in mildly sensitive people, the same is true of washing delayed for an hour. Under average field conditions, then, washing has little practical value. Similarly, little benefit is obtained from the use of tincture of green soap or other soaps based on alcohol or similar solvents.

In general, barrier creams offer no practical degree of protection against the dermatitis. Careful tests have proved that silicone creams, widely promoted about a decade ago, are valueless in preventing poison ivy dermatitis.

Dr. Kligman has conducted many tests with a galaxy of chemicals claimed to abort or prevent poison ivy dermatitis when applied to the skin after exposure or after the first blisters appear. Since poison ivy dermatitis is caused by a chemical, it seemed logical to try to neutralize this chemical with another. Many substances have been suggested, and many of them do indeed react with the chemical that causes poison ivy — but this does not mean they inactivate it. In fact, none of the chemicals tested had the desired effect. Dr. Kligman points out that the allergic process would be under way within an hour or two, perhaps irreversibly, even if it were possible to inactivate the poison ivy material still on the skin.

One of the ineffective chemicals Dr. Kligman tested was zirconium, for which enthusiastic — and groundless — claims have been made. At least eight OTC products used in the treatment of poison ivy dermatitis (including the popular *Rhulihist* lotion and its cream and spray counterparts) contain zirconium. Moreover, in addition to being ineffective, zirconium may be harmful. Even in minute quantities, this ingredient may cause granulomas — small, hard, painless lumps in the skin — in susceptible persons. Granulomas may take as long as eight to ten weeks to develop following application of a zirconium-containing preparation, and many zirconium-sensitive individuals (and often their doctors) do not associate the appearance of granulomas with earlier use of a zirconium-containing poison ivy remedy (or with an antiperspirant or deodorant — see Chapter 16).

For many years, physicians have used extracts of poison ivy, either orally or by injection, to build up immunity prior to exposure. In a special report to *The Medical Letter*, Dr. Kligman summarized his experience with methods of poison ivy "desensitization." He pointed out that "Complete desensitization of highly sensitive persons is not possible with *any* dosage. All that can be expected is a *reduction* in sensitivity (briefer, less generalized, less intense attacks in that order)." However, any reduction in the severity of symptoms can be a blessing to the sufferer. According to Dr. Kligman, intramuscular injections for desensitization are not really practical in clinical practice; too many injections are required, and even with conservative dosage adverse side reactions are numerous and may be severe. Dr. Kligman recommends oral dosage with a potent poison ivy extract (*Rhus* oleoresin) if treatment is undertaken.

In a long series of tests using a panel of five highly sensitive subjects, Dr. Kligman studied the effects of about thirty-four preparations. Not one medication tested was clearly more effective than tap water compresses and "shake" lotions containing a soothing ingredient such as zinc oxide or calamine. Antihistamines appeared to have no value taken by mouth or in ointments and lotions; ointments and lotions could even cause their own allergic reactions on top of the poison ivy eruption. Corticosteroid creams, ointments, or lotions, although they have many enthusiastic supporters, proved of no benefit in Dr. Kligman's controlled tests.

When the eruption affects a large part of the body, corticosteroid hormones taken under the care of a physician, either by mouth or by injection (in contrast to external application of creams or ointments), may benefit most severely affected patients within a matter of days. Such therapy usually lasts only a week or two, and therefore carries few of the well-known hazards of prolonged cortisone usage (see Chapter 27).

The widespread faith, even among some physicians, in poison ivy remedies that fail to stand up under controlled tests is probably a direct result of the fickle nature of the eruption. Its duration may vary markedly for no apparent reason, and the treatment being used generally gets the credit when the course is brief.

Most OTC products for poison ivy overmedicate. Almost all contain varying combinations of topical anesthetics, antihistamines, and antiseptics. Not only do these ingredients fail to relieve the discomfort of poison ivy, but they are also capable of adding to the discomfort by causing an allergic reaction. CU's medical consultants believe that none of these OTC combination preparations has been shown to be superior to ordinary calamine lotion. Therefore they recommend that anyone with a mild case of poison ivy use the cheapest brand available of ordinary calamine lotion, apply compresses of cool tap water, and take aspirin to help soothe the suffering.

For severe itching, however, compresses of very hot water (120° or 130°F) — hot enough to redden the skin temporarily — may relieve discomfort for as long as several hours. CU's medical consultants suggest that you try such treatment only when the poison ivy is localized in several small areas of the skin.

Chapter 14

Products
for
sun worshipers

SUNTAN AS A STATUS SYMBOL is a fairly recent phenomenon. For centuries the sun used to mark field hands and other outdoor laborers as members of the working classes, while the rich treasured their fair skin. In the years following the industrial revolution, when the poor left the sun to grow pale in factories, a suntan gradually came to distinguish those who could afford the luxury of sun year-round. Despite warnings in recent years that excessive sun can damage the skin — and even cause skin cancer — a suntan may still be sought in some circles, but it cannot be justified on grounds of health. Basking in the sun does not contribute to the well-being of the sunbather. Even the production of vitamin D, caused by the action of ultraviolet (UV) light on a certain chemical in the skin, requires only minimal exposure to sunlight.

Sunburn is the symptom of immediate sun damage to the skin. Although there is certainly a statistical basis for saying that more sandy-haired, light-skinned, blue-eyed people tend to experience this symptom than their dark-haired, olive-skinned, brown-eyed beachmates, the generalization may not hold for each individual. In checking the susceptibility to sunburn of volunteer subjects in a test of sunscreen products, CU found that dark-skinned individuals were not necessarily resistant to sunburn, and that freckled blonds were not necessarily extravulnerable.

How long you can remain in the sun without being burned depends on the thickness of your skin and its melanin content. (A pigment found in the epidermis, the uppermost layer of the skin, melanin is a genetically acquired characteristic.) It may also depend on whether you use a good sunscreen product (see below).

The major problem with sunburn is the cumulative effect of chronic damage. Over a period of years excessive exposure to the sun results in premature aging of the skin. This is manifested in many fair-skinned people by the eventual appearance on the exposed portions of the skin of wartlike growths (actinic keratoses) and of skin cancer. Darker-complexioned individuals, whose genetic inheritance has enabled them to produce more melanin than the fair-skinned, tend instead to develop thick, leathery, wrinkled skin. And those with heavier deposits of melanin, as is the case with blacks, rarely develop skin cancer or other signs of chronic sun exposure.

Countless vacations have been spoiled by overenthusiastic sunbathing on the first day. And the advent of the three-day weekend has brought more people than ever out into the sun, expecting to cram their suntanning into those precious few days. Even if fun in the sun is limited to weekends and vacations, most sunbathers can prevent both immediate agony and later unsightly peeling with judicious doses of caution and a good sunscreen preparation.

Both suntan and sunburn are caused by the invisible UV portion of the sun's spectrum. The amount of UV energy reaching a sunbather is affected by many things. The earth's atmosphere filters out some UV, so that a burn is more likely at higher altitudes where the atmosphere is thinner. This fact also explains why the sun's angle in the sky affects the burning potential; the skin burns fastest around midday (between 10:00

A.M. and 2:00 P.M.) and, some authorities believe, during the weeks just before and just after the summer solstice.

Other atmospheric conditions also affect the intensity of the UV rays that reach the skin. Because air pollution — a common ingredient in the skies of large urban centers — can obstruct passage of UV rays, sunbathing on the roof of a large city apartment building cannot be equated to sunbathing under the clear skies of a vacation spa. Similarly, haze and fog also filter out UV — but less than one might expect. Many sunbathers are badly burned on lightly overcast days when they mistakenly believe they are shaded from the sun.

And finally, UV rays, like visible light, are scattered by the sky, by light clouds, or by fog, and are reflected from surrounding surfaces. Green grass and water reflect relatively little UV; white sand reflects about 20 percent, while fresh snow can reflect as much as 85 percent. In some circumstances reflected UV (supplemented by the refracted and diffused rays of the sun) can be intense enough to burn those with susceptible skin even when they sit for several hours under an umbrella or an awning, sheltered from direct sunlight.

The first time out in strong sun after a stretch indoors, you should be cautious. If you tend to burn fast and badly, the first exposure of unprotected skin is safest early in the morning or in midafternoon. Others can begin closer to midday but, for safety's sake, it is wise to spend no more than a quarter-hour in the sun the first time. On subsequent days, extend your exposure by quarter-hour increments. If you use an effective sunscreen, you can substantially prolong your safe time in the sun.

However, tanning cannot be rushed. Too much sun at one time only burns the skin. If you insist on tanning, the safest way is simply to go out every day and stay no longer than the maximum recommended time. For those types of skin containing less melanin, tanning will remain an impossible dream. If you cannot tan, no product applied to the skin can help you.

You should know before you place too much faith in any sunscreen that all such products contain chemicals to which a few people are sensitive. Before using a new preparation, try it on a small area of the skin. If the skin does not redden or itch in twenty-four hours, there is little likelihood that an allergic reaction will occur. Nonetheless, use of any product should be halted immediately if the skin shows irritation, even if you have used the product safely before.

Almost all current commercial sunscreen products, whether sold as a lotion, cream, jelly, or aerosol foam or spray, contain chemicals that screen out skin-burning portions of the UV spectrum. But some products mistakenly used as sunburn preventives (baby oil, olive oil, and mineral oil, for example) do not have any special screening properties. Such products do not offer any protection against sunburn.

Careful application of the sunscreen preparation to all areas of exposed skin is essential. Protection can be increased by heavier application of the product. But dermatologists warn that if a greasy cream covers too much of the body surface at a time it may interfere with sweating and predispose to heat stroke. Also, an oily or greasy preparation can lead to boils and aggravate some skin disorders by blocking the sweat or sebaceous glands.

Perspiration, swimming, and rubbing by sand, towels, or clothing tend to remove any sunscreen preparation; the film of cream or lotion must be replenished from time to time. And for maximum safety, the preparation should be reapplied after each swim.

The suntan products currently on the market vary widely in their ability to protect against sunburn. In 1971 CU tested thirty-three of them, including lotions, creams, gels, butters, clear liquids, and aerosol foams; all screened out some UV, but none gave full protection to everybody. CU found, however, that the highest-rated brands (*Sungard, Estée Lauder Ultra-*

143

Violet Screening Creme, and *Irma Shorell's*) gave considerably better protection than the poorest ones. In the second-highest group were *Avon Sun Safe*, *Avon Bronze Glory Tanning Gel*, *Swedish Tanning Secret Extra Protection Lotion*, and *Sunstop by Bronztan*. However, even the less effective screens are useful for people who are not too susceptible to burning and for those willing to limit their early exposure to the sun. If through experimentation you find a particular product works well for you, be sure to match the name exactly when you go to buy it again; many companies make several suntan products with similar names but dissimilar performances.

One group of sunscreens that merits serious consideration includes those employing para-aminobenzoic acid (PABA) as the main ingredient. This family of sunscreens first came to wide attention in 1969 with publication of the results of a three-year study conducted by several researchers from the Harvard Medical School. More than 300 subjects were exposed to varying climatic conditions when covered with a wide variety of sunscreens, both laboratory-concocted and commercially available. Results showed that 5 percent PABA in 70 to 95 percent ethyl alcohol was distinctly superior to the other sunscreens tested, both in preventing sunburn and in resisting removal by swimming or excessive perspiration.

The Medical Letter has confirmed the value of PABA and has termed it "an excellent sunscreen" which can provide protection from sunburn and still resist loss of effectiveness through sweating. Commercial preparations using PABA include *Parafilm*, *Pabanol*, and *PreSun*. These products cost about $2.50 for 4 ounces. It may be possible to save some money by having your pharmacist prepare a sunscreen based on a version of the commercial formulation: 5 percent PABA in a solution of 50 percent alcohol, 30 percent water, and 20 percent glycerine. CU's medical consultants suggest that you check the cost with your pharmacist; the price may vary, depending on the availability of some ingredients. Formulas based on chemical modifications of PABA are used in *Block Out* and *Sea & Ski*, but do not offer as effective or as durable protection for the sunbather.

Another sunscreen of proven effectiveness is red veterinary petrolatum (RVP), an ointment now available over the counter (OTC) from Elder, the manufacturer of *Pabanol*. Of particular usefulness to those who may be sensitive to any of the commercial sunscreens are the products based on benzophenones (diphenylketones). These include *Uval* and *Solbar*, both available at drugstores. *The Medical Letter* warns, however, that these formulations are more vulnerable to sweat and bathing, and presumably need to be renewed more frequently.

For especially vulnerable areas, such as the nose and lips, a product that is a sunshade, rather than a sunscreen, may be necessary. Several OTC preparations are marketed for this purpose, but you can achieve the same result with a tube of zinc oxide ointment, available at a pharmacy.

Sun worshipers are targets for the promotion of less desirable products as well as useful ones. Perhaps the most curious of the sun-worshiper products are the chemical tanners which in 1960 became one of the hottest items in the drug trade. Dozens of manufacturers entered this field. The same tanning chemical, dihydroxyacetone (DHA), was used by all of them. Besides its use in straight tanning products, the chemical was added to aftershave lotions, sunscreens, and moisturizing creams. The profusion of products ended with the decline of the fad, but a few of them are still around. In fact, in 1972 *QT*, a sunless skin tanner, was the second leading product in sales of suntan preparations.

There is no doubt that DHA does darken the skin, but one cannot be sure the result will be the golden, natural-looking tan the products promise. Fortunately, if results are poor, the color wears off in a few days. In some users, the skin may temporarily take on a yellowish tinge; in others, the tan may be orange in color or blotchy. Also, DHA may discolor hair and clothing, especially with repeated use, and, as some users may have found out the hard way, the tan produced by DHA does not protect the skin against sunburn. CU's medical consultants do not recommend the use of DHA; they consider it a nonessential product and are doubtful about its usefulness as a cosmetic.

For those who insist on acquiring a tan without sun, there is a device more effective than chemical tanners — a sunlamp. However, it is also much more expensive and more dangerous. The supposed health benefits of sunlamps are practically nonexistent for most people. UV exposure to the point of peeling may help in some cases of severe acne (see page 117), but there are other skin conditions that UV worsens. When the skin is not healthy, the use of a sunlamp without medical supervision is a risky business.

The most immediate danger of sunlamps is the possibility of a bad burn. And just like sunburn, the full severity does not show up until several hours after exposure. Care should be taken not to exceed the time limits recommended by the sunlamp manufacturer. If users do not know how susceptible to UV burn they are, they should start with the shortest exposure time at the greatest distance recommended. Since it is not unusual to fall asleep while under a lamp, it is best to use a timer that shuts off the lamp automatically. Failing that, be sure to set a kitchen timer or an alarm clock.

The eyes need special protection from UV rays. Precautions should always be taken — even if the manufacturer of a particular sunlamp does not suggest any. UV can penetrate the skin of the eyelids and inflame the whites of the eyes; gross overexposure can even cause cataracts.

Anyone who spends much time in the sun ought to wear sunglasses. For maximum comfort the glasses should be dark, transmitting no more than about one-third of the visible light and, in bright sunlight, preferably no more than 15 to 20 percent. In addition, they should block most of the invisible infrared heat rays and the UV tanning rays, both of which in heavy doses can cause eye discomfort.

The sunglass lenses should be free of distorting imperfections which may disturb the sharpness of vision or contribute to eye fatigue. A shopper may find it helpful to hold the lenses a foot or two in front of the eyes and focus through the lenses on some geometric pattern. The design as seen through the lenses should not appear distorted or warped, even when the lenses are moved an inch or two up and down or side to side. Judging from tests made by CU several years ago, a large number of sunglasses on the market has been deficient in this respect. Fortunately, less-than-perfect sunglasses are unlikely to harm the eyes, although they may cause eye discomfort or slight headaches with prolonged wearing.

Plastic and glass lenses both come in high quality finely surfaced models and in inexpensive models with some surface ripples. Plastic lenses tend to scratch more easily than glass lenses, but they may be more protective against accidental flying debris. Most sunglasses are gray, green, or tan, although some are made in such colors as yellow, rose, or blue. Distortion of traffic lights or of any color tone is least with neutral lenses; CU tests found gray lenses the most neutral. No matter what color you choose, compare the two lenses to make sure they are equally dark.

Some high-fashion frames are so weirdly distorted that they allow too much light to filter in around the edges of the lenses. They may also be hazardous if they cut off peripheral vision. You can judge the quality of the frame by making sure there is no gap between the lens and the frame and no movement of the lens in the frame. The frame should have metal rather than plastic hinges with five or seven (not three) barrels and a screw fastener rather than a pin fastener.

Sun reflectors, widely advertised as an aid to year-round backyard tanning, can also sometimes prove hazardous to seekers of the sun. Typical of these products are metal face tanners (about $5) and silvered cushions (about $30). Dermatologists have warned that, if sun reflectors are used repeatedly for long periods of time, intensified UV rays can damage the skin. Used with moderation — and a good sunscreen — sun reflectors can be relatively safe for dedicated sun worshipers, especially those who practice their rites in late winter and early spring, when UV rays can do less damage.

A person using prescription drugs should check with a doctor before exposure to the sun or before using a sunlamp, because a wide variety of drugs taken by mouth can cause increased vulnerability to UV radiation. Such a reaction is called photosensitization (see Chapter 16). The trouble may show up either as a burn or as an allergic skin lesion, and can result in pain and severe discomfort from blistering. Notable photosensitizing agents include certain broad-spectrum antibiotics, (democycline, doxycycline, tetracycline), as well as a frequently used urinary antibiotic, nalidixic acid (NegGram). Griseofulvin (Fulvicin), an oral antifungal agent, and certain diuretics, such as chlorothiazide (Diuril), may also photosensitize. One of the major tranquilizers, chlorpromazine (Thorazine), has similar capabilities.

Sunscreens, despite the protection they offer against sunburn, do not always prevent possible photosensitivity reactions caused by drugs. Different chemical agents, including the drugs named above, sensitize the skin to other wavelengths in the UV spectrum than those against which typical sunscreens protect.

Chapter 15

The mouth odor fallacy

CHRONIC BAD BREATH (halitosis) is a symptom, not a disease. As with many symptoms, there are several possible causes, few of which are affected by *Colgate 100, Lavoris, Listerine,* or other mouthwashes, sprays, drops, tablets, toothpastes, and so on. Many odors are the result of mouth conditions — poor oral hygiene, decayed teeth, throat infections, canker sores, pyorrhea (see Chapter 5), postnasal drip, and the like. Such problems are easily detectable, and they need not, if handled correctly, result in mouth odors.

The fear of "offending" by means of mouth odor is apparently strong in our society. Many Americans (perhaps those whose "best friends" told them) develop the mouthwash habit. Sales of mouthwashes and gargles amounted to more than $260 million in 1975.

Most people notice a disagreeable taste and breath odor upon awakening. This is probably due to bacteria acting on food particles in the mouth during sleep. When a person is awake, bacteria and food particles are regularly dislodged by means of chewing, swallowing, and talking — as well as by random and purposeful tongue movements. During sleep these natural defenses are quiescent. But proper brushing or flossing of the teeth, or dental irrigation, before retiring does much to lessen the likelihood of a "brown" morning taste by removing the debris on which bacteria tend to multiply. Antiseptic mouthwashes might have some effect on the number of bacteria in the mouth, but these effects are transitory. The mouth regains its normal complement of bacteria within a short period of time. Although a mouthwash can also help wash away some of the debris, plain water can do it just as well.

Most mouthwashes contain alcohol. Regular use of such products may cause excessive drying of the mucous membranes of the oral cavity and may aggravate preexisting inflammation or infection. CU's medical consultants advise that, if you must use a mouthwash, select one without alcohol or one with a minimal alcohol content. The amount of alcohol in some brands of mouthwash ranges as high as 70 percent (*Astring-O-Sol*) and 61 percent (*Dalidyne*). Some of the better known brands, together with their alcohol content, are: *Listerine*, 25 percent; *Extra-Strength Micrin*, 20 percent; *Scope*, 18.5 percent; *Colgate 100*, 14 percent; *Cepacol* and McKesson's *Mouthwash and Gargle*, 14 percent; and *Lavoris*, 5 percent.

The ineffectiveness of commercial mouthwashes in combatting halitosis was underlined by the action of the Food and Drug Administration in 1970. This agency no longer permits manufacturers to claim that mouthwashes have any therapeutic value (see Chapter 4), even in regard to bad breath. Current promotion of these products centers on "freshening" the breath — a temporary effect, at best.

A bad taste in the mouth does not necessarily mean bad breath. And a person with a sweet mouth taste can have bad breath. A coated tongue may or may not be associated with a bad taste, bad breath, or both. True halitosis occurs most often without changes in the tongue or taste.

The pronounced although temporary odor that foods containing garlic, onion, and the like give to the breath does not originate in the mouth. It is caused by aromatic material absorbed from the intestine into the bloodstream, carried to the lungs, and then exhaled. Only a small proportion of garlic or onion odor is due to retention of particles in the mouth or between the teeth. Rinsing the mouth may wash away a few particles but has no effect on the major reason for the odor, which may take many hours to disappear. Smokers may also have a characteristic breath odor that mouthwashing does not correct.

Within recent years mouth sprays and drops have also been marketed. These products impart a pleasing fragrance to the breath — long enough perhaps for that good-night kiss, but not for much more. The only possible social benefit to be obtained from mouthwashes, drops, or sprays is the temporary replacement, with a nonoffensive aroma, of a bad odor that might be present. The same is true of the candy mints claimed to freshen the breath by absorbing odors. No substance is known that, in quantities that could be incorporated into a piece of candy, can absorb enough odor to solve permanently the problem of chronic halitosis.

Chapter 16

Banishing body odor

RESEARCH HAS SHOWN that sweat is not the culprit in the production of body odor. Rather, it is the interaction of sweat with the bacteria normally present on the skin that results in characteristic body odors. Three types of glands in the skin produce the secretions called sweat. Dermatologists generally believe that normal secretions of all three types of glands are odorless, or nearly so, until the secretions are decomposed by bacteria. The potential for odor formation is different for each type of gland.

The major source of body perspiration, the eccrine glands, are relatively unimportant in odor formation because eccrine sweat has only trace amounts of organic material on which bacteria can act. These glands help primarily to control the body temperature and, for the most part, are active only during exercise, in response to nervous tension or embarrassment, or when the environmental temperature is high. In certain areas of the body, such as the palms, soles, and axillae (underarms), they produce perspiration at lower temperatures and may become particularly active as the result of emotional stress. In some individuals, certain foods, especially "hot" spices, cause some of the eccrine sweat glands to become active.

Apocrine glands, in contrast, produce perspiration that is rich in organic material for bacterial action. Moreover, these glands are concentrated in the axillae, around the nipples, and in the genital area, the first and last regions being ideal sites for bacterial growth, not only because considerable perspiration occurs there, but because moisture cannot readily evaporate. Apocrine glands become active after puberty and remain so as long as sexual activity continues. There is also some evidence, not conclusive, that in women the activity of the apocrines may vary with the menstrual cycle. These glands are stimulated by emotional stress, such as fear or pain, and especially by sexual excitement; their activity is not increased by hot weather or by exercise.

Sebaceous glands, the third type of skin gland, lubricate the skin with an oily material called sebum (see page 110). They play a relatively minor role in the body odor of people who bathe regularly.

In view of what is known about the origin of body odor, there are two obvious approaches to its prevention: impede bacterial action, and reduce sweating. Deodorant soaps and deodorants are intended to accomplish the former; antiperspirants may do both.

Some antiperspirants are called deodorants by their manufacturers, but these products generally include a statement such as "checks perspiration" somewhere on their labels. The active ingredients of antiperspirants *must* be listed, because these products affect a body function (sweating) and are therefore considered *drugs* under the provisions of the Food, Drug, and Cosmetic Act.

Deodorant soaps and underarm deodorants, which are considered cosmetics under federal law, currently can be marketed with or without listing their active ingredients. The Food and Drug Administration (FDA) has announced that any cosmetic manufactured after November 30, 1976, *must* include information about ingredients on the product label. Until then, however, any body odor preventive that does not show a list of ingredients can be assumed to be a simple deodorant. But even if a product *does* list ingredients, it could still be a deodorant rather than an antiperspirant. Consumers can be sure it is an antiperspirant they are buying if they see on the label any claims about controlling perspiration or if they recognize one of the ingredients to be an antiperspirant agent (see below).

There can be little doubt that regular daily washing is the primary means of controlling both bacterial growth on the skin and body odor. Ordinary soap and water reduce odor by physically washing away bacteria and glandular secretions. Such soap is only mildly bactericidal. In recent years, antiseptics have been added to several brands of soap. These agents can help to reduce skin bacterial counts through daily use. One controlled study has demonstrated a statistically significant decrease in bacterial skin infections in users of soap containing hexachlorophene. But corroborative studies have been few.

In September 1972 the FDA announced that hexachlorophene would no longer be permitted in over-the-counter (OTC) preparations. An advisory panel on antimicrobial drugs recommended the action to the FDA on the basis of data impugning the safety of hexachlorophene. Studies using both animals and humans had demonstrated that unregulated routine use of hexachlorophene could be considered unsafe. Microscopic abnormalities in brain tissue of newborns had apparently resulted from the absorption of this compound into the blood through intact skin. Additional impetus to ban the antibacterial agent came after more than thirty French babies died from the application of a talcum powder contaminated with substantial quantities of hexachlorophene.

Serious questions continue to be raised about the safety of other antibacterial agents in deodorant soaps. After the ruling on hexachlorophene, production and shipment of soaps that included it were halted; hexachlorophene products are now available only on prescription. Many of the soaps later returned under the same brand name but reformulated by their manufacturers using other antiseptics, such as trichlorocarbanilide (or triclocarban) — called TCC — (used in *Dial*) and tribromosalicylanilide — called TBS.

According to reports stemming from the same panel of doctors who initiated the ban on hexachlorophene, panel members were not very happy with the substitutes either. In their opinion, these chemicals, like hexachlorophene, were also risky because, in significant amounts, they too could be absorbed through the skin. And, the panelists noted, the amounts of these chemicals that can be safely used in a lifetime have not yet been established. When the antimicrobial panel studying soaps and skin cleansers submitted its final report to the FDA in September 1974, panel members suggested prohibiting the nonprescription use of TBS.

Some dermatologists have even called for a warning label to be printed on deodorant soaps. Their concern has also centered around the fact that some of the newer antiseptics are photosensitizing agents, thus raising the possibility that someone using such a deodorant soap may experience a severe reaction when exposed to sunlight. In some instances, blistering skin reactions have led to hospitalization; such patients sometimes have to avoid sunlight for indefinite periods. Less severe cases can be successfully treated with corticosteroids and temporary avoidance of sunlight. TBS, which has been implicated as a photosensitizing agent, was at one time used in a number of deodorant soaps including *Irish Spring, Lifebuoy, Phase III, Safeguard,* and *Zest.*

Unlike ordinary sunburn, a photosensitivity reaction can involve considerable swelling and blistering (rather than peeling). It is not unusual for reactions to occur even after three weeks have elapsed between initial contact with the deodorant soap and subsequent exposure to sunlight. With continued use of the offending product, however, the incubation period can become much shorter. And the use of a sunscreen may not always protect against a photoallergic reaction (see page 148).

It is well to view with skepticism any advertising claims for antibacterial soaps. In August 1973 the Federal Trade Commission (FTC) made public the test data submitted by various manufacturers of soaps and detergents to substantiate claims made in promotion of their products. It turned out that both Procter & Gamble and Armour-Dial had hired "trained judges" who tested deodorant soaps by "actually sniffing each armpit to ascertain which product provides better odor control" and then rated the products on a scale of zero to ten. The sniffers from Procter & Gamble found *Safeguard* the best protector against "offensive odor," while Armour-Dial's sniffers found *Dial* soap at least as effective as *Safeguard*.

Particularly worthy of skepticism are any claims that the routine use of antiseptic soaps will prevent boils and other infections of the skin. People with recurrent skin infections or boils should check with their physicians. Some diseases such as diabetes may have skin infections as their only overt symptom.

Although soaps containing antiseptic agents can effectively reduce the number of skin bacteria and thus possibly diminish body odor, CU's medical consultants are opposed to their use unless recommended by a physician. In any case, it is probably possible to obtain longer-lasting protection against bacteria in the underarm area with a deodorant containing an antiseptic than with soap containing an antiseptic, because more of the deodorant chemical remains on the skin.

The simple application of a deodorant, however, cannot remove bacteria or any previously decomposed material. Such an application is not a substitute for bathing, and should follow adequate cleansing of the area. A few deodorants depend mainly on odor substitution, their perfume temporarily masking a disagreeable odor with one that is more pleasant.

Several years ago, chlorophyll was widely promoted as the

answer to all odor problems. It was included in "bad-breath" tablets, mouthwashes, toothpastes, skin preparations, and dog foods — even impregnated into clothing. Consumers spent tens of millions of dollars on chlorophyll products, but it is now clear that chlorophyll has no regular or lasting effect on either body or mouth odor.

It has been suggested that neomycin and other antibiotics, in skin preparations, can effectively control underarm odor by inhibiting bacterial growth. Although somewhat effective, such preparations may induce allergic reactions in some individuals, or encourage development of strains of microorganisms resistant to the antibiotics (see Chapter 28). Revlon's *Hi & Dri* cream and roll-on and *Top Brass* roll-on contain neomycin, and Gillette's *Right Guard Deodorant* lists "antibacterial agents" among its active ingredients. CU's medical consultants advise consumers to shy away from such products.

Many antiperspirants contain some type of aluminum or zinc salts such as aluminum chloride, aluminum sulfate, aluminum chlorohydroxide complex, basic aluminum formate, aluminum phenolsulfonate, or aluminum sulfamate. Like the antiseptics used in deodorants, these salts retard bacterial multiplication. In addition, they reduce the amount of sweat that reaches the skin surface. How they do this is not definitely known, and the effectiveness may vary from person to person and from time to time in a given individual. It is possible that these antiperspirants control one type of perspiration more effectively than another, for example, perspiration due to hot weather (eccrine glands) better than that due to emotional stress (eccrine and apocrine glands), or vice versa.

One notable exception — while it lasted — to the standard formulations was *Mennen E*. This product, manufactured by the Mennen Company, attempted to ride the tide of the vitamin E fad (see Chapter 21), but distribution was halted in May 1973 because of complaints of allergic skin reactions made to the

FDA by people who had used *Mennen E* deodorant.

According to its maker, *Mennen E* exploited the alleged anti-oxidant nature of vitamin E. The theory was that vitamin E inhibits bacteria from utilizing oxygen to break down under-arm secretion into odorous substances. From the number of letters received by the FDA telling of allergic reactions, including severe rashes, some consumers apparently got more than they expected from the use of *Mennen E*. Although shipments of the product were discontinued, the FDA permitted remaining stocks of *Mennen E* to stay on the shelves. CU's medical consultants suggest that consumers do likewise.

Antiperspirants currently on the market are relatively useless for a small group of people who have a condition known as hyperhidrosis, an abnormality involving the production of a large amount of sweat by the underarm glands and also at times by the glands of the hands and feet. No entirely satisfactory solution is known. This kind of abnormal sweating is thought to be due to localized overactivity of the sympathetic nervous system. Medications are usually of no help; in rare instances surgery may be required.

At times excessive sweating is an appropriate response to emotional stress or physical exercise. Excessive perspiration of the feet may produce a particularly objectionable odor because of the action of bacteria on the superficial skin layers of the soles. In addition, retained sweat on the feet encourages the growth of fungi, which cause acute and chronic inflammations such as athlete's foot. People whose feet perspire excessively should, whenever possible, wear sandals or open-weave shoes, and hose of cotton or wool rather than nylon or silk. Liberal dusting of the feet with plain talc helps absorb sweat and discourages growth of fungi. Lamb's wool tucked between the toes keeps them apart and aids in the evaporation of perspiration.

Several years ago, the aluminum salts used in antiperspirants were quite acid. As a result, they sometimes irritated the skin of the armpit and stained and weakened clothing fabrics. Present-day products are rarely sufficiently acid to damage fabrics; they seldom irritate the skin — except momentarily, perhaps, if applied too soon after shaving. Allergic dermatitis from aluminum salts is also rare, but anyone who experiences significant irritation should avoid the preparation that seems to cause it. In switching brands be sure that you choose one with a different active ingredient. A product with the simplest formula may be the least likely to cause reactions.

In the past, some users of antiperspirants containing a zirconium salt developed granulomas — tiny, hard, painless, long-lasting lumps in the skin — in their armpits. Zirconium salts are no longer added to the formulations of most antiperspirants. Current exceptions are Procter & Gamble's *Secret* and *Sure* roll-on and cream products. The aerosol spray versions of *Secret* and *Sure* were reformulated in mid-1976 to eliminate zirconium. However, Dr. W. L. Epstein, Professor of Dermatology at the University of California Medical Center, reports that granulomas have not been observed to any measurable degree in experimentally sensitized people tested with *Secret*.

In October 1973 the Gillette Company announced withdrawal of two new antiperspirants with a formulation identified on the label as an aluminum zirconyl hydroxychloride complex. Both *Right Guard Extra Strength Anti-Perspirant* and *Soft & Dri Extra Strength Anti-Perspirant* had been marketed for less than a month. Unlike other *Right Guard* and *Soft & Dri* products, these versions contained zirconium. The antiperspirants were reported to have caused a mild lung inflammation in monkeys used in safety tests.

By way of recapitulation, it is clear — despite the ads — that no deodorant or antiperspirant is a substitute for washing. Some people who do not perspire much may find that regular bathing is all they need. Although a deodorant soap may help, its

159

continued use may lead to an unpleasant, and sometimes permanent, photosensitivity reaction. An antiperspirant is probably a better selection than a simple deodorant, since it does all that a deodorant does and reduces perspiration as well. Most people find one of the aluminum salt antiperspirants satisfactory, although it may be necessary to try several brands to tell which is most effective for you.

No matter which brand you select, be sure to buy the product in the form of a roll-on, cream, lotion, or stick — and not as an aerosol. CU's medical consultants warn that prolonged and repeated exposure to aerosol sprays can be potentially harmful (see page 311).

Depend on your own comparison shopping to make the best choice, and not on the ads. The FTC has shown some interest in advertising claims made for nine products representing about 80 percent of the estimated $460 million annual market for antiperspirants and deodorants. For example, in May 1973 the FTC declared it wanted to be told, "in plain language" understandable to the average consumer, what the basis is for claims by *Right Guard* that it has "the best wetness fighter . . ." or by *Soft & Dri* that the product doesn't sting "even when used right after shaving." Also requested was supporting research data for the boast by the makers of *Ultra Ban* that their product keeps people drier than any leading spray. In November 1973 the FTC asked for substantiation of advertised claims for five more antiperspirants and deodorants. In July 1975 the FTC put on the record the documentation submitted in support of the claims. It now remains to be seen whether consumers will encounter more modest claims and less flamboyant language in magazine ads and television commercials, for which the makers of these products spend about $40 million a year.

Chapter 17

Genital deodorants for women

IN THE 1960s the cosmetic industry realized that its valiant — and profitable — campaign to ban body odor could be extended beyond the underarm area. By 1966 the genital deodorant was ready for its commercial debut; soon corner drugstores were displaying rows of genital deodorant sprays for women (and even brands for men). The age of the genital cosmetic flowered, and by 1971 there were thirty brands of "feminine hygiene spray" (the euphemism for women's genital deodorants) for which Americans were willing to spend $67,710,000.

A typical feminine deodorant spray nowadays includes an emollient acting as a carrier, a propellant, and a perfume. No one can be positive about the ingredients because under present law a "cosmetic" product need not list all — or any — of its ingredients on the label. After November 30, 1976, however, the Food and Drug Administration (FDA) will enforce a requirement that labels for newly manufactured cosmetics include information about ingredients (see page 169). Until September 1972, when the FDA banned use of hexachlorophene in over-the-counter products, many formulations included hexachlorophene. However, most manufacturers of genital sprays never replaced the banned chemical with other antibacterial agents.

Even today, when consumers have become less frightened of

genital "odor" and more informed about the hazards of the product, sales figures indicate the business is still lucrative. In 1975, the total spent on genital deodorants was $20,320,000 — the drop undoubtedly reflecting the record of painful injuries, discomfort, and irritations attributed to use of the product.

Another probable factor in the sales dip was the influence of women who resisted the sales pitch. For example, Germaine Greer, author of *The Female Eunuch*, dismissed the deodorants with the comment that she had never seen anyone lying around overcome by vaginal fumes. Other leaders of the women's liberation movement joined in condemning the vaginal spray as a totally useless and demeaning product. Dr. Natalie Shainiss, a New York psychiatrist, said at a Senate hearing in 1971, "While fostering an overt message of a feminine, 'sexy' woman, the implication of need for such a spray conveys a message of woman as being dirty and smelly — extremely damaging to a woman's sense of self."

The initial sales success of genital deodorants can be attributed to more than the American preoccupation with how we smell to one another or increasingly relaxed attitudes towards sex. Madison Avenue's ability to create a market also played a part. The uninhibited advertising for genital cosmetics reflected the ingenuity of copywriters in selling the wares of their new clients. According to many of the advertisements, genital sprays not only enhance a woman's sex appeal, but they also keep her from being downright offensive.

In a college issue of *Mademoiselle*, Roycemore's *Demure* cautioned: "You don't sleep with Teddy Bears anymore." Warner-Lambert's *Pristeen* genital spray warned, "Unfortunately, the trickiest deodorant problem a girl has *isn't* under her pretty little arms." The Personal Products' division of Johnson & Johnson advertised its female genital spray, *Vespré*, as "the intimate odor preventive." ("Some sprays hide it. Some sprays mask it, but *Vespré* actually prevents intimate odor.")

Television advertising for genital deodorants alone reached an annual rate of $10 million by 1971. In typical Madison Avenue style, the demand had been created for a new product. "In this world of accelerating change, new ideas and new products are constantly originated that contribute to the betterment of our lives and broadening of our horizons," reported the president of Alberto-Culver, manufacturer of *FDS* (a leading product in the field).

Dr. Bernard A. Davis, a Montreal gynecologist, was less enthusiastic about this latest contribution to the full life. He reported treating about thirty cases of inflammation of the genital area following the use of feminine sprays. "Surely," he said, "in this gadget-conscious, product-oriented civilization, we must resist those instances where a demand is being artificially created for a product of questionable value. This is especially true where even the minimal advantage can be more than outweighed by significant complications."

The president of Alberto-Culver said in defense of female genital deodorants that they solve a problem dating from biblical times. The "problem," as seen from the manufacturer's vantage point, is as old as woman herself. The external genitals, the vulva, contain glands capable of producing mildly odorous secretions. Close-fitting underwear, pantyhose, or tight slacks tend to delay evaporation of perspiration. Normal skin bacteria act on those secretions and produce an odor which the cosmetic industry would have women regard as unpleasant.

To the extent that those vulval odors occur naturally, as they do to a greater or lesser degree in most healthy women, CU's medical consultants advise soap and water as the most effective and certainly the safest hygiene. And *The Medical Letter* states, "It is unlikely that commercial feminine hygiene sprays are as effective as soap and water in promoting a hygienic and odor-free external genital surface."

Many vaginal infections give rise to foul-smelling vaginal discharges. Less commonly, an unsuspected tumor of the uterus or cervix may produce secretions which are also malodorous. Under pressure from advertising about her "tricky" deodorant problem, a woman might be persuaded to disguise these pathologically caused odors by masking them with a perfumed deodorant spray.

However, some odors may be due to the presence of a foreign body, such as a forgotten tampon or contraceptive device. Or menstrual flow may occasionally be accompanied by malodor. Soap and water does not take care of odors from these causes. But neither does a chemical spray. Indeed, the use of a genital deodorant may discourage some people from washing often enough. And most important, CU's medical consultants are concerned that the use of genital sprays may make some women with medically significant odorous discharges put off seeking medical advice while using the sprays instead.

Advertising, moreover, may suggest that genital deodorants should be sprayed directly into the vagina instead of onto the *external* genital area. Such internal use could be especially dangerous. According to Dr. Bernard M. Kaye, a gynecologist and assistant professor at the Abraham Lincoln School of Medicine of the University of Illinois, "There is an implication of vaginal use in the names of the products and the advertising. Vaginal use is absolutely contraindicated and will lead to irritation from the propellant and/or the ingredients of the product."

Again as a result of advertising, women may believe that the moment prior to sexual intercourse is the ideal time to make use of this "cosmetic" product. CU's medical consultants warn that it is particularly ill-advised to apply a female genital deodorant just before intercourse because there is the chance that the freshly sprayed chemicals might be carried into the vagina. Moreover, according to *Today's Health*, an American Medical Association publication, there have been reports of male genital irritation attributable to intercourse with a partner who had used a genital spray deodorant immediately before.

In a letter to *The New England Journal of Medicine* in July 1972, Dr. John M. Gowdy of the FDA's food division, which has jurisdiction over cosmetics, reported that a variety of complaints about genital deodorant sprays had been received by his agency, and noted, "The offending ingredient has not been identified." Dr. Gowdy stated that, although the reactions were not life-threatening, "all were locally severe, and average recovery time was thirty days." Dr. Gowdy added that pressure from propellants "may be important" in setting up local inflammation of the urethra (the short passage from the bladder to the outside).

Such inflammations may result in narrowing of the urethra, which not only can cause painful urination but, more importantly, can lead to consequent retention of urine within the bladder. This in turn leads to recurrent urinary tract infections, which, as many women know, can be troublesome and difficult to cure with medication, and may sometimes require dilatation of the urethra or other surgical treatment.

In January 1972 CONSUMER REPORTS published an article on genital deodorants, describing them as potentially hazardous, and documenting its case with reports of injuries and serious harm. (Because these products had been classified as "cosmetics," rather than drugs, they escaped the extensive premarketing test programs required of all new drugs to establish their safety and effectiveness.) It was some time before the FDA took any action. Finally, in June 1973, more than a year after CU first broke the story on the dangers in using genital sprays, the FDA proposed that a mandatory warning be required on every package. The FDA also took note of the misleading "hygiene" or "hygienic" usually tacked on the descriptions of these products, and denied manufacturers the right to use such terminology with its implication of medical benefit. However, the FDA did not reclassify genital sprays as drugs but permitted them to remain in the cosmetic category and thus to continue to be sold to consumers who might not read the warnings on the label. (As of this writing, the FDA expects products manufactured after November 30, 1976, to carry new labels.)

Most authorities would go further than the mandatory warning the FDA has proposed for these products. Even the FDA's own advisory panel of obstetricians and gynecologists voted unanimously in October 1972 that genital deodorants should be considered drugs and therefore made subject to extensive controlled testing for safety and effectiveness before further marketing would be permitted. The FDA warning, intended "to minimize any possible risk to users," does take one very minimal step to deal with possible hazards to users. It includes a recommendation that the spray be kept at least 8 inches from the skin; some products on the druggists' shelves still suggest "about 6 inches." Unfortunately, CU does not know of any genital deodorant that comes packaged with a ruler.

Although many people may be able to use genital deodorants without apparent ill effect, there is always a risk involved in applying chemicals to the body, especially to such sensitive areas as the genitals. (Indeed, there is an additional hazard in the prolonged and repeated use of aerosol sprays — see page 311.) But manufacturers of genital deodorants tend to shrug off any possible risk as insignificant. Warner-Lambert, the makers of *Pristeen*, and Alberto-Culver say they receive adverse reactions at a rate of only six per million sales. Even at that rate, as of April 1971 Alberto-Culver had reports of 107 women users of *FDS* who had complained of irritation, allergic reactions, burns, infection, dermatitis of the thighs, stinging, swelling, itching, inflammation, a lump, and even a burned hand. (The company had to furnish this information to a court in connection with a lawsuit filed by a woman who claimed to have been injured by *FDS*.)

The number of complaints probably understates the problem.

Most people, after all, do not bother to write; they merely stop using the product. A few may consult a doctor, and never suspect that the deodorant is the real cause of their discomfort. Dr. Kaye reported in a periodical, *Medical Aspects of Human Sexuality*, on interviews with his patients. Of twenty women questioned, fourteen said they had used a genital spray deodorant; of those fourteen, four reported vulval itching or burning.

Some reported cases went beyond mere discomfort. One fourteen-year-old girl was described by her physician as having suffered "incredibly" swollen labia. In one of at least two lawsuits filed against Alberto-Culver, a woman who used *FDS* spray alleged that she quickly developed large lumps and had to be admitted to a hospital when the condition became so painful that she had difficulty walking. Her doctor diagnosed the problem as a severe reaction to *FDS* spray. "The swelling was as big as a grapefruit," her physician said. "You never saw a more miserable girl in your life." Her lawsuit against Alberto-Culver was settled out of court.

When a college student wrote to Alberto-Culver asking about the risk of adverse reactions to *FDS* spray, the company told her, "While the occurrence of such reactions is rare compared to the number of people who use the products regularly, they do occasionally occur and can be quite painful." The firm called attention to its label directions instructing the user to hold the can about 6 inches from the body while spraying. Then it added some information not found on the label: "Holding the spray too close might deposit a concentrated amount of the spray on the body and this could cause some irritation."

In view of such possibilities, what kind of safety testing was done before the genital deodorant was brought to the market?

An indication of the type of testing necessary was supplied in a technical article by John A. Cella, Ph.D., Alberto-Culver Vice-President for Consumer Product Research, in the October 1971 issue of *American Perfumer and Cosmetics.* "In formulating deodorant products, as with all toiletries, sufficient testing should be done *in vitro* [sic] in animals and humans to assure that the product is safe for repeated use and is effective in delivering the label claims," he wrote. According to Dr. Cella, "minimum testing" for a female genital spray "should include animal skin irritation and sensitization studies, animal vulvar irritation studies, animal vaginal instillation studies using the aerosol concentrates, human repeated insult patch tests on intact and abraded skin, subacute and chronic human use tests, particle size analysis of the spray and animal inhalation studies." Dr. Cella also called for extensive laboratory and use tests to determine the effectiveness of female genital sprays.

Despite Dr. Cella's call for extensive safety testing, Alberto-Culver's sworn pretrial statement in the aforementioned lawsuit did *not* include most of his test proposals when it outlined the testing done prior to the marketing of *FDS* in 1966. Furthermore, an FDA medical officer who reviewed the Alberto-Culver data disagreed sharply with the company's conclusions and stated: "Thus while close to 25 percent of the subjects seemed to have some type of adverse reaction to the product, the company reports no irritation or other abnormality."

In 1971 in response to a questionnaire from CU, Alberto-Culver listed several tests it claimed to have conducted *after* introducing *FDS* on the market. However, they hardly compensated for the totally inadequate premarket test program set forth in the pretrial testimony. Had the FDA agreed to reclassify female genital sprays as drugs — instead of merely requiring that a warning label be affixed — manufacturers would have been required to provide evidence concerning the safety and effectiveness of their products. The nature of that evidence might prove embarrassing for the entire deodorant industry if Alberto-Culver's premarket test program was at all typical.

Problems of safety in using genital deodorants are part of the larger picture of cosmetics and their hazards. The best answer to these problems is stronger cosmetics legislation. A bill introduced by Senator Thomas Eagleton, the Cosmetic Safety Amendments of 1976, which passed the Senate in July 1976, would require premarket clearance by the FDA for all cosmetic products. Senator Eagleton plans to introduce similar legislation in the next Congress.

In June 1975 the FDA set regulations for the marketing of cosmetics labeled as "hypoallergenic." After June 6, 1977, all manufacturers would be required to submit evidence of clinical testing to substantiate claims that their products cause fewer adverse reactions in human subjects than competing brands.

Meanwhile, the FDA has proposed a partial solution to the problem of cosmetic labeling. In October 1973 the FDA issued regulations requiring ingredient labeling for all cosmetic products. Labels would have to list ingredients in descending order of predominance. The FDA ruling will take effect for newly manufactured cosmetic products after November 30, 1976. Consequently, as of this writing, there has still been no real change in cosmetic labeling, and until the FDA requirement for ingredient labeling is enforced after November 1976 — or until there are new rules or legislation is passed — people with allergies and those hypersensitive to certain chemicals will still be playing guessing games with the cosmetics they use.

The one cosmetic consumers can surely do without — even should all its ingredients be clearly marked on the label — is the genital spray deodorant.

Chapter 18

The quacks

QUACKERY THRIVES MOST in those areas of human illness for which there is no cure. When legitimate expertise fails, patients often turn to other sources. Whether in continuous pain, suffering from varying degrees of disability, or just experiencing vague discomfort, these patients may become prey to outright quacks, as well as to licensed doctors on the fringe of organized medicine. Both of these types promise relief from symptoms — for a price. They also sell hope. Self-styled health practitioners offer devices or nostrums; and some physicians offer an unjustified medical diagnosis, with an expensive "treatment" to match.

The commercialized promotion of products for serious illnesses has been profitable for the outright quacks, because they are fined, jailed, or enjoined from operating only when regulatory agencies have sufficient time, money, manpower, and incentive to carry through the years of litigation often required. It has been estimated that quackery costs Americans more than $2 billion annually. No one knows how many people have died of cancer because they relied on quackery until the disease had advanced too far for orthodox medical treatment to be of help; nor how many elderly arthritics have dissipated their life savings chasing one false hope after another (see Chapter 19); nor how many diabetics have had tragic setbacks after abandoning reliable therapy for some worthless nostrum.

There are, of course, federal, state, and local laws intended to protect the public from the deception that causes so much disappointment, as well as wasted time and money. But enforcement against even the most flagrant offenders is difficult. State and local enforcement agencies are generally so poorly staffed that they can act only infrequently; and when they do, the offender often merely pays a fine (if any) and moves the operation elsewhere. The brunt of the enforcement load, then, is carried by three federal agencies, each of which has a more-or-less circumscribed area of authority and all of which have a heavy load of other responsibilities for their limited staffs: the Federal Trade Commission (FTC), the Food and Drug Administration (FDA), and the U.S. Postal Service.

The FTC has authority to act against false and misleading advertising of over-the-counter preparations; the product (or the advertising) first must move in interstate commerce, however. Until recently the mechanics of FTC action allowed for so much legal maneuvering that it often took years to halt misleading advertising. Only after the maneuvering was all over and the offender subsequently violated a cease and desist order could the FTC take the case to court to impose any kind of penalty at all.

In 1973 Congress gave the FTC authority to seek an injunction to halt unfair or deceptive acts or practices. The FTC used its new powers to obtain from a Federal Court in January 1974 an order barring three travel agencies from advertising and promoting "psychic surgery" tours to the Philippines. The tour participants — mainly people with serious or terminal illnesses who had given up on conventional medical care — were offered "spiritual healing," a process by which a person's body is supposedly entered without cutting to remove diseased tissue. The court authorized the FTC to notify the people who had signed up for such tours that " 'psychic surgery' . . . is not an actual surgical operation, no incision is made, and diseased tissue is not removed from the human body."

The FDA has authority for action (1) if products are misbranded, (2) if there are false or misleading claims in the labeling (which includes accompanying literature such as leaflets or pamphlets) of a food, drug, cosmetic, or medical device sold in interstate commerce, (3) if products are dangerous, or — in the case of drugs — ineffective, and (4) if new products are sold before they have complied with premarket procedures enforced by the FDA. Under any of these conditions, the FDA may request that the attorney general seize shipments of the product and hold them until a federal court determines their disposition. The FDA may also request that the attorney general institute criminal action against the shippers of such products.

In testifying before a Senate subcommittee in February 1974, the FDA commissioner listed "a number of deficiencies" in the Food, Drug, and Cosmetic Act. The commissioner recommended passage of legislation that would broaden the agency's factory inspection powers, give it subpoena authority comparable to that already exercised by the FTC, and provide for speedy and effective enforcement. Under the present system, products that may be violating the law are subject to seizure only after application to the courts. "We have found, however, that on a number of occasions a suspected product has been shipped before seizure can be accomplished," the commissioner explained, in requesting the power of administrative seizure.

The Postal Service has authority to act against anyone who uses the mail to defraud or with intent to defraud; proving a violation in court, however, has not always been easy. The Postal Service's authority to deal with quackery has recently been increased. It now has the power to seize or impound merchandise before final disposition of a case, including the period when appeals might be pending. Representatives of the American Medical Association (AMA) report that the Postal Service has been using this power to deal with mail-order sales of questionable medical devices and materials.

One might suppose that the three agencies together could do a reasonably good job of policing quackery. In practice, however, it turns out to be very difficult to stop a determined peddler of questionable medical products or services. One case history, in which all three agencies had a hand, is illustrative.

Back in 1919 the Post Office Department issued a fraud order against Jesse A. Case of Brockton, Massachusetts, the promoter of a once-famous remedy called *Case's Rheumatic Specific*. Thereupon Jesse A. Case filed an affidavit stating that the sale of this rheumatism remedy had been discontinued and that it would not be revived.

Not long afterward Jesse's son, Paul Case, announced a new treatment for rheumatism, said to be based on a "prescription" received from a "noted French physician," one Dr. Beaupré. "The prescription cost me nothing," Paul Case's ad declared. "I ask nothing for it. I will mail it to you if you send me your address." And he was as good as his word.

Those who answered the ad did receive a free copy of the "prescription." By a curious coincidence, as the *Journal of the American Medical Association* pointed out in 1924, "this marvelous treatment . . . is strikingly similar to the . . . treatment exploited by . . . Jesse A. Case, before the Government interfered." But Paul Case's prescription contained an additional ingredient — a substance called powdered gadoeng, imported from Java. Your corner drugstore could hardly have been expected to carry powdered gadoeng in stock; and so Paul Case had made arrangements to offer a thirty-day supply for $4.

In 1933 the FTC brought a complaint against Paul Case for falsely representing that his product — now named the *Case Combination Treatment* but no longer containing powdered

173

gadoeng — would "drive out aches and pains of muscular and sub-acute rheumatism, neuralgia, gout, sciatica, neuritis, and lumbago." Case defended himself, but in January 1934 he was ordered to cease and desist.

In July 1938 the FTC again checked up on Case; he was still selling a rheumatism remedy. In 1942 he was still at it — and the FTC brought a second complaint. This one was heard in 1944. Case explained that he had added aspirin to his formula. Despite this addition, the FTC in October 1947 again ordered him to cease and desist from making excessive claims.

In 1939 and again in 1946, the Post Office Department considered taking action against the Paul Case rheumatism remedies, but took no action on either occasion. In 1947 the FDA brought criminal charges against Case in connection with claims for a tonic he was also peddling. Case pleaded guilty to this charge, and in March 1948 was fined $250. So far as CU has been able to determine, this was the only actual penalty ever assessed against him.

What had been accomplished, in short, by the whole series of FDA, FTC, and Post Office Department proceedings from 1919 on, was little more than to take the color, flamboyance, and verve out of the Case sales material.

The delays, the switch in operations, the repeated offenses, and the lack of significant penalty encountered with the Cases are not just isolated episodes. In 1959 the FTC finally completed a sixteen-year campaign to have the word "liver" removed from *Carter's Little* [Liver] *Pills*. The FDA spent ten years trying to halt the sale of the Hoxsey cancer treatment. In December 1960 the FDA announced that "The Taylor Clinic [successor to the Hoxsey Clinic previously closed] has completed the final step required by a Federal court injunction prohibiting distribution of treatment." But twice in 1961 new announcements came of seizures of the Taylor treatment. The first announcement was linked with notice of a consent decree against a seller of another worthless cancer cure, the Koch treatment, the peddling of which had theoretically been stamped out in 1958. Still other "cancer cures" have come in for FDA investigation and action.

Quackery can often take a much more simple — and tragic — form. A recent example of misplaced religious fervor was the death in August 1973 of an eleven-year-old diabetic whose parents refused to continue his insulin treatment after they were convinced by a faith healer that their son was "cured." Faith healers do not always bring death; more frequently they just take your money. A health food store proprietor reported to *The New York Times* in 1973 that he collected $7 a visit from customers who submitted to painful foot massage to "loosen tensions" and send a stream of oxygen through the body. The "treatment" brought health, happiness, and long life. When supplemented by the purchase of certain health foods (for $40), the "treatment" also improved the customer's sex life and relieved any chronic diseases.

An absorbing account of how this kind of charlatanism has persisted in our age of scientific enlightenment may be found in *The Medical Messiahs — A Social History of Health Quackery in Twentieth Century America*, by James Harvey Young. First published in 1968 by Princeton University Press, this 460-page book is currently available to the readers of CONSUMER REPORTS in a CU paperbound edition.

The AMA, whose Bureau of Investigation has been a clearinghouse for information about quacks and quackery for fifty years, has suggested certain guidelines for spotting a quack. Beware, it warns, if self-styled medical experts use a special or secret machine or formula they claim can cure disease; if they guarantee a quick cure; if they advertise or use case histories and testimonials to promote their cures; if they clamor constantly for medical investigation and recognition; if they claim representatives of organized medicine are persecuting them or are afraid of their competition; or if they tell you that surgery, X rays, or drugs will cause more harm than good.

If, after applying these rules, you still have doubts about a treatment or cure suggested to you by an advertisement, a book, a friend or a relative, you can obtain helpful answers to questions from a variety of public service organizations. (Most of these organizations appreciate being notified of questionable activity in their areas of special interest.) Some of the reliable places to try are:

The Food and Drug Administration District Offices, as listed under Health, Education, and Welfare Department in telephone directories of the cities where they are located, or its national office, Rockville, Md. 20852.

The Federal Trade Commission, Bureau of Consumer Protection, Washington, D.C. 20580.

The U.S. Postal Service, 1200 Pennsylvania Avenue, N.W., Washington, D.C. 20260 – for information and complaints about mail-order products.

The Consumer Product Safety Commission, Bethesda, Md. 20016.

The American Medical Association, Bureau of Investigation, 535 North Dearborn Street, Chicago, Ill. 60610.

The American Cancer Society, The Unproven Methods of Cancer Management Committee, 777 Third Avenue, New York, N.Y. 10017.

The Arthritis Foundation, Room 240, 475 Riverside Drive, New York, N.Y. 10027.

Council of Better Business Bureaus, Inc., 845 Third Avenue, New York, N.Y. 10022.

Your state or local health department, medical society, or food and drug enforcement agency.

The vigor shown by the AMA in pursuing outright quacks has not been matched by equal energy and diligence in unmasking questionable practitioners who operate under the cloak of official licensure. In this area the AMA has been virtually derelict. Although machinery exists for depriving physicians who are incompetents or charlatans of their right to practice medicine, the procedures are so cumbersome that they are seldom invoked. The authority to hear charges and, theoretically, to revoke licenses is delegated to state and county medical societies. These bodies are usually content merely to reprimand a physician brought up on charges. The physician, duly reprimanded, is then permitted to resume normal practice.

This kind of wrist slapping does little to upgrade the quality of medical care. The traditional image of the doctor as an inviolate guardian of health care has changed in recent years more because of the misconduct of a few physicians than because of any pervasive flaw in the medical profession as a whole. CU believes that more stringent penalties for abuses of medical privilege are needed, as well as more responsibility on the part of state and county medical societies (see Chapter 31).

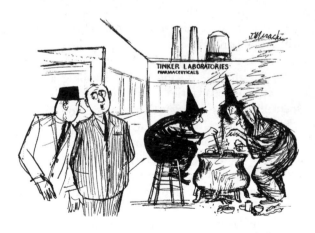

"We figure they may hit on something."

Chapter 19

The mistreatment
of arthritis

AN ESTIMATED TWENTY MILLION AMERICANS suffer from some arthritic disability; millions more experience minor symptoms. These people, who constitute America's biggest market for quack remedies, spend perhaps $400 million a year on misrepresented arthritis treatments or "cures."

According to The Arthritis Foundation, the names "arthritis" and "rheumatism" are used popularly for about 100 ailments characterized by pain in the joints and muscles. Of these ailments, by far the most common are osteoarthritis and rheumatoid arthritis. The latter is one of a group of diseases that affect the connective tissues of the body. Rheumatoid arthritis tends to be a recurring process during which swelling and, in some instances, eventual deformities occur in many joints of the body, especially in the hands. Women are more commonly affected than men; the ratio is 3 to 1. The disease usually starts between the ages of twenty and forty-five, but may occur in children. With this disease characteristic changes occur in the blood, frequently including the appearance of a protein, called "the rheumatoid factor," which can be detected by a specific test. Osteoarthritis is best described as a "wear-and-tear" disease in which the large weight-bearing joints (such as the hips and knees) are most frequently involved. Other joints and the fingers may also be affected. Some authorities believe the disease to be a part of the aging process, since it is seldom experienced before the late fifties.

Neither osteoarthritis nor rheumatoid arthritis is now curable, although medical treatment can usually relieve symptoms, may prevent or postpone disability, and in many cases can modify disability already caused by the disease. Both disorders are subject to periods of remission in which pain spontaneously subsides and — in rheumatoid arthritis, particularly — all disease symptoms seem to disappear. If a period of improvement happens to coincide with the use of a remedy, the patient may well be convinced that the remedy "cured" the disease. This is the basis for many sincere testimonials for worthless products.

It would be hard to find any type of quack treatment that has not been promoted for arthritis. And sufferers from arthritic disorders are apparently good customers. Mailing lists of arthritics are used over and over; once patients have sent their names and addresses to a single advertiser, they are likely to receive mail about a whole string of products.

The Arthritis Foundation classifies current mistreatments into four principal groups: advertised clinics, devices, diet fads, and drugs and other medications. In addition to mistreatments, there is also the category of misleading publications.

ADVERTISED CLINICS

Many clinics, some of them associated with springs and spas, advertise treatment for arthritis. Some of the theories advocated in the sales literature of these clinics and spas (such as the theory, for example, that arthritis is caused by constipation or toxemia) were discarded by doctors years ago. The lure of some so-called arthritis clinics in Mexico and Canada is of growing concern. In addition to advocating costly treatments not in accordance with accepted theories, these clinics dispense large quantities of potentially harmful drugs, which are brought

179

back into the United States for unsupervised use. A new twist has been added by some Mexican clinics — "information centers" based in the United States, and designed to recruit patients for over-the-border treatment. CU's medical consultants warn potential clients of such clinics to be skeptical of any unorthodox treatment for arthritis.

DEVICES

Among the most popular devices are vibrators; an example was the *Pulse-A-Rhythm* vibrating mattress, seized by the Food and Drug Administration (FDA) along with literature making therapeutic claims. Vibrators are ineffective in treating arthritis, and they may be dangerous in the acute phases of rheumatoid arthritis.

Uranium has been widely promoted; an arthritic can buy mitts or pads filled with low-grade ore. (Or the patient can pay for the privilege of sitting in an abandoned uranium mine to absorb the "healing radiations.") Fortunately, the amount of radiation, where investigated, has been found to be minute; but even minute amounts of radiation may induce cumulative effects which could be harmful.

In a special category are pulsating diathermy machines, which have been heralded in newspaper publicity as "a dramatic breakthrough in the treatment of arthritis." There is no medically substantiated evidence that such devices have any advantage over the ordinary diathermy apparatus physicians sometimes use as part of a program of therapy.

There are also various questionable diagnostic machines touted to arthritics. One such machine, the *Micro-Dynameter*, was the subject of nationwide seizure by the FDA following a court decision. The FDA called it "a peril to public health." Evidence introduced at the trial included readings given by the *Micro-Dynameter* that showed no difference between a corpse and a living person.

DIET FADS

Sellers of many food supplements and proponents of offbeat diets include arthritis in the long list of ailments supposedly helped by their products or by their dietary regimens. But there are no medical findings supporting the use of any sort of special food or diet in treating arthritis. Alfalfa, pokeberries, and, for that matter, vitamin and mineral supplements have never been shown to be effective.

DRUGS AND MEDICATIONS

No matter how persuasively disguised, most over-the-counter (OTC) products promoted for use by arthritics have aspirin or some other OTC analgesic as their chief ingredient. Often this is not stated in the advertising. *Anacin,* for example, claims that "the pain medication doctors prescribe most for arthritis also has a most effective anti-inflammatory action. What you should know is that this same medication is in today's *Anacin* tablets." What you should also know — and you can find it out by reading the package label — is that *Anacin's* two active ingredients are aspirin and caffeine. The caffeine is a holdover from *Anacin's* old formula based on a USP formulation for *A.P.C.* tablets; it was kept — presumably for promotional purposes, since there is no rational therapeutic reason for caffeine being included — when *Anacin* dropped phenacetin as an ingredient (see Chapter 1). True, the aspirin in *Anacin* does suppress inflammation, but at several times the cost of plain aspirin tablets, which suppress it just as well.

Three new arthritis-oriented analgesic products have now appeared on the market. The first, *Arthritis Pain Formula* analgesic tablets, is alleged "by the makers of *Anacin*" to provide "extra medication and extra protection." A tablet "contains 7½ grains of microfined Aspirin" instead of 5 grains of "large, rough, jagged particles" of "regular" aspirin, plus two antacids (aluminum hydroxide and magnesium hydroxide). The second, *Arthritis Strength Bufferin*, provides a dose of aspirin 50 percent larger than that in regular *Bufferin* — 7.5 grains versus 5 grains — along with increased amounts of two antacids. The third, *Bayer Timed-Release Aspirin*, contains double the aspirin in an ordinary *Bayer Aspirin* tablet. In general, timed-release preparations are unreliable with regard to their absorption into the bloodstream (see page 36); also, side effects, when they occur, tend to be prolonged.

To the degree that aspirin in these "arthritis products" happens to meet the requirements of an arthritic's disorder, they may bring a measure of relief, but it is expensive relief. Plain aspirin costs a lot less. The average patient with active rheumatoid arthritis who tolerates aspirin may be maintained on as many as twenty 5-grain tablets of aspirin a day. When one considers such therapy in terms of months or years, the cost mounts up. Even more important, the patient who relies on "arthritis products" instead of consulting a doctor loses the chance for additional relief from pain or for protection from disablement that medical care can often provide.

Liniments, ointments, and body rubs are heavily promoted for the relief of aches and pains due to arthritis. These OTC products depend on one or more skin irritants for their effect. *Ben-Gay Pain-Relieving Ointment* uses methyl salicylate (oil of wintergreen) and menthol; *Deep Strength Arthritis Pain Relief Rub* (*Musterole* in a special formulation) adds camphor to these ingredients. *Heet Spray* goes one step further and adds a fourth irritant, methyl nicotinate; *Heet Liniment* uses a different formulation, but still sticks with methyl salicylate as one of the ingredients. Both *Exocaine* and *Ger-O-Foam Aerosol* list methyl salicylate as their only irritant, but add an anesthetic, benzocaine, to their aerosol spray formulation. (For a warning against the possible hazards of using aerosol spray products in the home, see page 311.)

Unfortunately, most manufacturers persist in treating their formulations as "trade secrets" and refuse to provide the necessary quantitative information that might help the arthritic make a rational choice of a drug. Of thirty-three external analgesics listed in the *Handbook of Non-Prescription Drugs*, six contain no methyl salicylate and rely on other irritants. Of the twenty-seven products that use methyl salicylate, ten do not give any quantitative information. And the quantitative information given for the remaining seventeen offers little reassurance. The concentrations of methyl salicylate range as high as 20 percent for *Mentholatum Deep Heating Lotion*, 30 percent for *Ger-O-Foam Aerosol*, and 50 percent for *Panalgesic*. *Sloan's Balm* (2 percent) and *Sloan's Liniment* (2.7 percent) contain the least amount of methyl salicylate.

Application of these external analgesics tends to increase blood flow in the upper layers of the skin, resulting in a slight reddening of the skin as well as a sensation of warmth. This mild increase in skin temperature may provide symptomatic relief for a brief period.

However, CU's medical consultants warn against the indiscriminate use of external analgesics with high methyl salicylate content (see above). According to *The Pharmacological Basis of Therapeutics*, edited by Drs. Louis S. Goodman and Alfred Gilman, absorption of methyl salicylate can occur through the skin and can result in systemic toxicity. Absorption is speeded up if the drug is applied to mucous membrane or to areas where the skin is cut or inflamed. The use for children of preparations containing this drug should be strongly discouraged.

A note of caution to the user of any external analgesic: A heating pad should never be used in conjunction with a liniment or external analgesic. Severe burns with blistering may result.

The small victory of the Federal Trade Commission (FTC) in its effort to tone down the advertising of *RU-EX Com-*

pound, an OTC product depending on a salicylate, shows how difficult it is for government agencies to give consumers any lasting protection from these products. *RU-EX* advertising used to be headed: "Lemon juice recipe checks rheumatic and arthritis pain." The FTC ordered the company to stop claiming that lemon juice, however used, exerts any therapeutic effect on arthritis. The words "lemon flavor" were substituted for "lemon juice" in the heading, and similar small changes were made in the text. Thus the ruling was "obeyed" with, one would guess, little detriment to sales.

Government regulatory agencies were confronted with a far more serious problem in dealing with the arthritis "remedy," *Liefcort.* That story was given wide circulation in an article entitled, "New Arthritis Controversy," in the May 22, 1962, issue of *Look* magazine. It told of a home-brewed hormone remedy created by Robert E. Liefmann, a then unlicensed doctor in Canada who wanted to do a favor for an arthritic friend. "I just went downstairs and mixed it up," Dr. Liefmann is quoted as saying. "By God, I hit it right on the head." He claimed *Liefcort* "could practically wipe out the symptoms of arthritis in one year," and prescribed it for any arthritic who happened to come by.

Without giving his remedy the usual preliminary tests for safety (or revealing its ingredients), Dr. Liefmann tried to have it tested clinically. Medical investigators refused to dose patients with an untested secret remedy; Dr. Liefmann went directly to the press. A Canadian newspaper ran the first article, and then *Look* spread the word across the United States. American arthritics began to stream across the border to pay Dr. Liefmann $9 per ounce for *Liefcort.*

As with every arthritis "remedy," many were ready to swear to its effectiveness. But soon there were also reports of side reactions, particularly abnormal uterine bleeding. In October 1962, after a California woman died of pneumonia following an operation to halt such bleeding, the FDA issued a warning and began to seize *Liefcort* at the border. The FDA denounced the drug as "imminently dangerous," and prohibited its importation into the United States. Canada banned the use of *Liefcort* in clinical investigations.

Samples of the drug obtained and analyzed in 1962, and again in 1968, revealed the main ingredients to be varying amounts of a corticosteroid, prednisone, plus male and female hormones (testosterone and estradiol, respectively). All three drugs have been used for years, separately or in combination, in treating some cases of arthritis and certain other diseases. Because of serious side effects, these hormones must be prescribed and used with great care.

In 1962 Dr. Liefmann obtained a license to practice medicine in Canada, and established a clinic in Montreal. On May 1, 1968, his license was suspended for five years for permitting unauthorized persons to practice medicine in his office. He filed an appeal, however, which had the legal effect of restoring his license. But on May 2, 1968, the Canadian government seized "all available supplies" of Dr. Liefmann's drugs; he was then charged with sixteen violations of the Food and Drugs Act. In June, according to the *Montreal Gazette*, the doctor had boosted the price of *Liefcort* to $30 per ounce, and was advising patients to "stock up." The newspaper reported that "patients must buy a six-ounce quantity — or nothing. This means that men pay $180 while the women — who receive two bottles — pay $360." In September of 1969 Dr. Liefmann was convicted on all counts and fined a total of $2,400. He died in 1972 with the case still under appeal. However, clinics in both Canada and Mexico continue to offer arthritis sufferers the "formula" concocted by Dr. Leifmann — and to reap the profits.

MISLEADING PUBLICATIONS

Many people tend to believe that something read in a newspaper or magazine, or in a book issued by a well-known publisher, is true. "They" must have checked or "they" wouldn't dare say it. There are, of course, many good publications on health problems; there are also many bad, although essentially harmless, ones; finally, there are a few that are actually dangerous.

In 1968 a paperback book called *Arthritis Discovery*, published without any listed author or editor, was offered for sale by mail in the United States and Canada. Subtitled *The Attempted Murder of Canadian Arthritis Discovery — The Crime Plotted by the Medical-Drug Cartel, Pseudo-Charity, Establishment*, it was "dedicated to the Robert Liefmann Clinic." The Arthritis Foundation calls the book "a reprehensible document calculated to induce more arthritis sufferers to go to Canada to obtain a contraband and dangerous drug." The book was revised and republished in 1971 under the title, *Arthritis Is Not Forever*.

Numerous other books on arthritis have been published over the years. Some play on the hopes of desperate arthritics, using such titles as *Arthritis Can Be Cured, Victory over Arthritis, There Is a Cure for Arthritis*, and *A Doctor's Proven New Home Cure for Arthritis*. Two other books — with less daring titles — have been read eagerly by some arthritics: *Arthritis and Folk Medicine* by D. C. Jarvis, M.D., and *Good Health and Common Sense* by Dan Dale Alexander, both published in 1960. These two books have another similarity: Each author has discovered *the* answer, the one real, true, right answer to the problem. Here the similarity ends, since each answer is quite different.

Although Dr. Jarvis is dead, his last book is not. As readers of his previous best-selling *Folk Medicine* would expect, in *Arthritis and Folk Medicine* he also advised the use of *Honegar*, a mixture of honey and vinegar, with additional doses of iodine and kelp. Dr. Jarvis cited no human case histories, but he told many stories of cows that were cured of milk fever, or produced better calves, or yielded more tender meat after slaughter, if vinegar had been poured on their rations.

Copies of Dr. Jarvis's first book were seized by the FDA in connection with sales of *Honegar*. But a book in itself cannot be seized because of false or misleading content; it must be sold in connection with a product to become subject to seizure by the FDA.

Unlike Dr. Jarvis, Dan Dale Alexander is not a medical doctor. As he tells the story, he was a schoolboy when be became interested in arthritis because his mother had it.

"I traveled to libraries throughout Connecticut, reading everything I could find on the topic of arthritis. I consulted medical textbooks, health magazines, technical publications — always searching for a clue."

He decided that diet was the answer, and his mother's condition "responded favorably" when she followed his rules. Despite the fact that he had no medical training and had done no clinical work, he evolved a theory that "differs from any other in the world." It has to do with such matters as avoiding water at meals, and drinking cod-liver oil with orange juice. Also, Mr. Alexander distinguishes between two kinds of sweets, two kinds of starches, and two kinds of oils.

At an FTC hearing on the promotion of Alexander's earlier book, *Arthritis and Common Sense*, the hearing examiner commented on "the impressive lack of medical or other training or education which would fit Alexander to write a book on such a recondite subject." Alexander and his publisher were ordered to stop advertising that the dietary regimen in the book was a reliable treatment or cure for arthritis. But the FTC could not prohibit sale of the book itself, nor could it prevent Alexander from writing and publishing his later book, in which the advice on arthritis remained about the same, although the advertising claims were much more moderate.

RECOMMENDED READING ON ARTHRITIS

Pamphlets on arthritis in general, and on specific subjects such as rheumatoid arthritis, osteoarthritis, gout, and home care, are available free — in quantity, at low prices — from The Arthritis Foundation, Room 240, 475 Riverside Drive, New York, New York 10027. Among its activities concerned with prevention and possible cure of arthritis, this agency supports clinics where patients can obtain treatment at costs geared to their ability to pay.

Readers interested in additional information on arthritis should consult the following books recommended by The Arthritis Foundation:

Arthritis: Complete Up-to-Date Facts for Patients and Their Families, Sheldon Blau, M.D., and Dodi Schultz (New York: Doubleday, 1974).

The Arthritis Handbook: A Patient's Manual on Arthritis, Rheumatism and Gout, Darrell C. Crain, M.D. (Hicksville, N.Y.: Exposition Press, 1971; 2nd ed., revised). Also available in paperback.

Beyond the Copper Bracelet: What You Should Know about Arthritis, Louis A. Healey, M.D., Kenneth R. Wilske, M.D., and Bob Hansen (Springfield, Ill.: Charles C Thomas, 1972). Out of print; available in paperback.

Living with Arthritis, A. B. Corrigan, M.B. (New York: Grosset & Dunlap, 1971). Out of print.

The Truth About Arthritis Care, John J. Calabro, M.D., and John Wykert (New York: David McKay, 1971).

Understanding Arthritis and Rheumatism: A Complete Guide to the Problems and Treatment, Malcolm I. V. Jayson, M.D., and Allan St. J. Dixon, M.D. (New York: Pantheon, 1975).

Chapter 20

Low blood sugar: fiction and fact

SOME AFFLICTIONS, such as arthritis and cancer, are so widespread or so painful that they become a fertile field for practitioners of magic "healing" who promote a grab bag of cures. Working the other side of the street are those who exploit patients with a variety of nonspecific symptoms by fitting them all neatly into a single diagnostic category. Hypoglycemia — or low blood sugar, as it is commonly called — is a perfect case in point.

Hypoglycemia is a real enough disorder, although relatively uncommon. In recent years, however, it has become the easy solution to a set of ill-defined complaints. As a result, the questionable diagnostic practices of a few doctors account for far more "victims" of hypoglycemia than do valid medical indications. These doctors have found it convenient — and profitable — to label patients hypoglycemic, sometimes without laboratory evidence to substantiate the diagnosis. And even when these doctors run proper diagnostic tests, they misinterpret — or ignore — the laboratory evidence.

A world of fiction has been created about hypoglycemia. For a variety of reasons, many people undergo periods in which they experience fatigue, insomnia, irritability, faintness, depression, and a host of other burdensome complaints. Few such people suffer from low blood sugar. Low blood sugar in and of itself — and unrelated to a specific physical disorder — is seldom responsible for such complaints. Nevertheless, a small number of determined physicians tends to attribute many of those emotional disorders and vague feelings of being unwell to low blood sugar. The treatment they prescribe consists of a low-carbohydrate diet and periodic injections of adrenal cortical extract (a relatively weak extract of hog and beef adrenals), generally referred to as ACE. These injections, of course, involve considerable expense to the patient.

The use of ACE in treating hypoglycemia is based on the notion that low blood sugar is always caused by inadequate secretion of certain hormones by the adrenal glands. The adrenals are best known for the manner in which they bring you to full alertness and energy in a crisis, but they also help to stabilize the level of blood sugar. (See Chapter 27 for a more detailed discussion of adrenal hormones and their actions.) Because of the connection between the adrenals and blood sugar, the Hypoglycemia Foundation, Inc., and those who adhere to its teachings, maintain that injections of ACE can increase the blood sugar level. They tend to associate most cases of low blood sugar with "tired" or "worn-out" adrenal glands.

According to CU's medical consultants, there is no evidence that adrenal insufficiency plays any role in functional hypoglycemia (see page 196), nor is there proof that ACE, used as recommended by the Hypoglycemia Foundation, would help, even if there were. CU's medical consultants know of no evidence, in the form of controlled clinical observations, that ACE has any place in the treatment of hypoglycemia — or for that matter in the treatment of any disease.

ACE has been on the market for more than forty years. It is now produced only by Parke, Davis — since Upjohn discontinued the product in August 1973 — as a treatment for chronic Addison's disease, a rare condition. According to CU's medical consultants, ACE is no longer recommended for this disease. *AMA Drug Evaluations* calls ACE "obsolete," and adds: "There is no known medical use of this drug."

The Food, Drug, and Cosmetic Act does not require the manufacturer of ACE or any other drug marketed prior to 1938 to demonstrate its effectiveness to the Food and Drug Administration (FDA). The FDA can control the sale of a pre-1938 drug only on the grounds that the drug is improperly labeled.

Treatment of hypoglycemia has not been among the uses of ACE indicated by Parke, Davis — or, before its discontinuance, by Upjohn. Indeed, if Parke, Davis were now to claim that ACE is an effective treatment for hypoglycemia, ACE would then be considered a new drug, the effectiveness and safety of which would then have to be demonstrated to the satisfaction of the FDA before it could be marketed.

There is no evidence to suggest that Parke, Davis has been promoting the use of ACE for hypoglycemia. The company acknowledges that such use "has not been approved by the FDA [and that] consequently, we do not suggest its use in this particular condition at this time."

Despite the relative infrequency of documented hypoglycemia, the disease has received widespread publicity in books and magazines. In 1971, a major article in the *Ladies' Home Journal* said that it affected "millions of Americans, particularly women between the ages of 25 and 50." From where does all this publicity come?

The Hypoglycemia Foundation is a low-budget, tax-exempt foundation headed by a board of directors of nine, of whom two are physicians; it operates from the suburban New York apartment of one of its officers. Its immediate goal "is to put recognition and treatment of hypoglycemia on a par with diabetes" and to alert physicians to hypoglycemia "and indoctrinate them in its proper treatment." Its publication, "Delinquent Glands Not Juvenile Delinquents," suggests that "a goodly percentage of juvenile delinquents would become happily well adjusted individuals if their hypoglycemia were recognized and treated." Another pamphlet advises that "controlling hypoglycemia is frequently relatively simple, and that such control could do much to prevent diabetes and to reduce alcoholism and drug addiction; to combat juvenile delinquency, mental retardation, chronic fatigue, asthma, allergies, and many other serious problems" (see illustration on page 199).

People apparently hear of the foundation by word of mouth or through a handful of widely sold books. One of these, *Goodbye Allergies*, has sold more than fifty thousand copies. Its author, Tom R. Blaine, an elderly Oklahoma judge, described himself as a "cured" hypoglycemic. His book portrays hypoglycemia as something of a modern-day black plague, and attributes many of mankind's problems to low blood sugar.

A foundation official, Marilyn Light, who learned about hypoglycemia from Judge Blaine's book and who claims to have been restored to full health by the diet and ACE treatment described therein, told CU in 1971 that about 300 physicians in 42 states and the District of Columbia were registered with the Hypoglycemia Foundation. Marilyn Light said most of those physicians had an average case load of 250 "hypoglycemia" patients. (A doctor in Salt Lake City was said to be treating 500 people.)

The fountainhead of much of the erroneous information disseminated by the Hypoglycemia Foundation and its several hundred physician-allies is the teachings of the late John Tintera, a Yonkers, New York, doctor. Dr. Tintera's involvement with hypoglycemia followed publication in 1951 of *Body, Mind and Sugar*, by Dr. E. M. Abrahamson and A. W. Pezet. The book, which has been frequently reprinted, attributes to low blood sugar a variety of mental and physical disorders said to affect about ten million Americans. This same condition, the authors claimed, is responsible "for the moral breakdown that underlies all delinquency and crime." The authors conceded that their views were not accepted by the medical profession, but that this was "largely because most doctors have not yet had time to read the literature." The treatment outlined by Dr. Abrahamson consisted primarily of a diet similar to that prescribed today by many physicians — a diet relatively low in carbohydrates with multiple feedings in place of the usual three meals.

Dr. Tintera, in a series of medical journal articles published in the late 1950s and early 1960s, went beyond Dr. Abrahamson by recommending the use of ACE to combat low blood sugar, to which he, like Dr. Abrahamson, attributed a frightening number of conditions, including fatigue, alcoholism, mental disorders, and allergies. In 1958 Dr. Tintera presented some of his views in a series of articles in *Woman's Day* magazine, causing his peers in the Westchester County (New York) Medical Society to call him to appear before it. The society's executive director told CU that Dr. Tintera had been censured for writing an article in a lay magazine on endocrinology, a subject in which he allegedly had no formal postgraduate medical training. Some time later, the society received a complaint from a young university professor who claimed that Dr. Tintera had given him weekly injections of ACE for seven months. Dr. Tintera allegedly told the young man that he would need the injections for the rest of his life. After having spent hundreds of dollars on ACE, the young man entered a hospital for a series of tests, which revealed no abnormalities. In 1967 the Westchester County Medical Society advised Dr. Tintera to abandon his treatment for hypoglycemia. But there is nothing to suggest that Dr. Tintera did abandon his particular brand of medicine prior to his death in 1969.

Aside from the mild rebuke to Dr. Tintera, CU found little

evidence until 1973 that the medical establishment has tried to crack down on physicians who practice medicine according to the recommendations of the Hypoglycemia Foundation. For example, after receiving a complaint about one of its members who was administering ACE for hypoglycemia, the Nassau County (New York) Medical Society contented itself with recommending that the doctor inform patients of the unorthodox nature of his treatment. The executive director of the society acknowledged that the organization had made no effort to ascertain whether the doctor has followed the society's recommendation.

What are the facts about hypoglycemia? The fictions flourishing in recent years moved CU to set the record straight in a July 1971 article in CONSUMER REPORTS. In January 1973 the medical establishment finally saw fit to comment on hypoglycemia. Three prominent organizations of physicians and scientists — the American Diabetes Association, the American Medical Association, and the Endocrine Society — issued a joint statement echoing the CU position. The organizations stated that "the majority of people" with symptoms of sweating, shakiness, trembling, anxiety, fast heart action, headache, hunger sensations, brief feelings of weakness, and, occasionally, seizures and coma "do not have hypoglycemia." The organizations then pointed out that a great many patients with anxiety reactions have symptoms of this kind. (It was seven months later, in August 1973, that Upjohn stopped manufacturing and distributing ACE, leaving Parke, Davis as sole producer.)

Reviewing the medical facts of the disorder, these organizations voiced the same judgment about ACE that CU had expressed in CONSUMER REPORTS two years earlier. Their joint statement said, in dismissing ACE, that "there is no known medical use for it. In fact, the few drug companies still manufacturing this preparation do not list treatment of hypoglycemia as one of its uses. Thus it should be stressed that administration of adrenal cortical extract is not an appropriate treatment for any cause of hypoglycemia." CU welcomed the statement and expressed the hope that it might signal some stirring within the medical profession to take effective action against doctors who persist in treating their patients with ACE. According to CU's medical consultants, if some of these patients feel better, their improvement is more likely due to diet and the power of suggestion than to ACE.

Now let's look at the facts about hypoglycemia. *Hypo* (low) *glycemia* (sugar in the blood) is not a disease, but rather a complex of symptoms. Nor is it a constant condition; almost invariably, attacks are episodic.

Under normal circumstances the level of sugar in the blood is maintained within certain limits by the opposing actions of different physiological forces. The blood sugar level in the body is increased either by eating foods containing sugar or by the release of sugar stored in the liver in the form of a complex carbohydrate, glycogen. Two potent hormones that cause the liver to release sugar are glucagon (made in the pancreas) and adrenaline (made in the adrenal glands). Counteracting those hormones is insulin, another hormone, manufactured in and released by the pancreas. Insulin facilitates the utilization of blood sugar by the various cells of the body, which then transform the sugar into energy. The normal stimulus to the release of insulin is an increase in blood sugar level.

When the blood sugar falls in rapid fashion to a significantly subnormal level, a surge of adrenaline is released from the adrenal glands as the body attempts to restore the low blood sugar to a normal level. The action of adrenaline on the glycogen stored in the liver causes this complex carbohydrate to break down and release sugar into the bloodstream, thereby restoring the normal blood sugar level. In the process, the rapid release of adrenaline also affects the heart and the nervous system, causing such symptoms as trembling, sweating, palpitations, nervousness, and headache.

A second variety of hypoglycemic symptoms is due to the direct effect of the low blood sugar itself on the functioning of the central nervous system. These symptoms usually occur at a blood sugar level lower than the level that triggers the adrenaline-release symptoms listed above, and are frequently preceded by them. More severe than those adrenaline-release symptoms, the second variety of hypoglycemic symptoms includes mental aberrations, personality changes, bizarre behavior, and even temporary amnesia. These abnormalities of central nervous system functioning tend to follow a repetitive pattern, each episode being characterized by the same set of abnormalities.

Any hypoglycemic episode can be dramatically relieved, although just temporarily, either by the ingestion or injection of glucose (sugar) or by an injection of glucagon.

By far the most frequent cause of a hypoglycemic reaction is an excess of insulin taken by a patient with diabetes mellitus. Other types of hypoglycemia can be divided into two categories: functional (reactive) hypoglycemia and organic (fasting) hypoglycemia. The functional type follows a meal — sometimes by as long as three to four hours. Organic hypoglycemia occurs in the fasting state, after eight to twelve hours without food. The more serious of the two, organic hypoglycemia may be characterized predominantly by the central nervous system symptoms described above (rather than the adrenaline-release symptoms). Organic hypoglycemia always requires intensive medical investigation and treatment.

Functional hypoglycemia is believed by some physicians to be due to the *excessive* production of insulin by the pancreas in response to an increase in blood sugar; the release of that excess insulin abruptly decreases the blood sugar to an abnormally low level, which brings on the hypoglycemic symptoms. In some cases of functional hypoglycemia, however, insulin release has been shown to be normal. Thus in some people the hypoglycemia may actually be due to an abnormal sensitivity to normal amounts of insulin. A diagnosis of functional hypoglycemia must be documented by a glucose tolerance test that is *definitely* abnormal.

A glucose tolerance test is always taken on an empty stomach. After a small amount of blood is withdrawn from the patient's arm, the patient drinks a measured amount of sugar solution. Blood samples are then taken at suitable intervals for four or five hours, and analyzed for sugar. The rate of rise and fall of blood sugar is studied, and deviations from normal standards are noted. (A more common form of the glucose tolerance test is the three-hour version, used primarily for the detection of diabetes mellitus, not hypoglycemia.)

During the course of a glucose tolerance test, the patient is observed for typical symptoms — the adrenaline-release symptoms mentioned earlier. Most physicians are aware that many normal people — those with no symptoms at all — have what appears at first glance to be a low blood sugar level during the course of the five-hour glucose tolerance test. Many authorities believe this to be an entirely normal phenomenon. In such instances, however, blood sugar rarely falls to less than 45 or 50 milligrams per 100 cubic centimeters of blood. In fact, CU's medical consultants emphasize that only when the blood sugar level falls below 45 milligrams per 100 cubic centimeters can it be said that hypoglycemia does indeed exist.

Relatively few people who complain of nervousness, anxiety, depression, palpitations, and so on, actually have functional hypoglycemia, according to CU's medical consultants. And those who do, often have severe emotional problems. Whether the symptoms are caused by emotional problems, or vice versa, has not yet been resolved. Most endocrinologists believe that many people with one type of functional hypoglycemia are prediabetic and will eventually develop diabetes mellitus, especially if there is a family history of the disease. Another type of functional hypoglycemia may be encountered in individuals who have had stomach operations for peptic ulcer.

Treatment for a diagnosed case of functional hypoglycemia generally consists of restricting carbohydrate intake. Standard low-carbohydrate (75–150 grams per day) diets are prescribed, and the number of daily meals is increased from the usual three to about five or six smaller ones. Carbohydrate restriction as treatment for functional hypoglycemia may seem contradictory, considering that glucose (a carbohydrate) is taken to relieve an acute attack. When used to relieve an attack, the sugar restores blood levels to normal, leading to easing of symptoms. When used as part of dietary treatment, however, sugar restriction can forestall the excessive release of insulin — and an attack of functional hypoglycemia.

Organic hypoglycemia is much more rare than the functional type. The organic type can usually be diagnosed by detection of a low blood sugar level after an overnight fast. The level of insulin in the blood may also be measured and, if found to be high, an insulin-producing pancreatic tumor is usually the likely suspect. Less commonly, other kinds of tumors produce insulinlike substances which act to lower the blood sugar level. In addition, advanced liver disease, congenital liver enzyme defects, chronic adrenal disease, or deficient pituitary function may also cause organic hypoglycemia. Tests that distinguish among these various causes are complicated, but are readily available. These tests are essential for selection of the proper therapy. If organic hypoglycemia is left untreated, or treated improperly, the symptoms of an attack could progress from adrenaline-release symptoms to central nervous system symptoms including convulsions, coma, and even death. Treatment of organic hypoglycemia consists of appropriate therapy for the underlying disease, such as surgical removal of the tumor.

CU's medical consultants emphasize that under no circum-

stances is ACE ever an appropriate treatment for any disease
— including, of course, hypoglycemia.

DO YOU HAVE ONE OR MORE OF THESE SYMPTOMS?
IT MAY BE   HYPOGLYCEMIA
-LOW BLOOD SUGAR-
Allergies--Exhaustion--Fatigue
Alcoholism-Dizziness-Drug Addiction
Poor Concentration-Irritability-Depression
Craving for Sweets-Caffiene-Nervous Breakdown
CHILDREN--under achievers or and Behavior Problems
FOR FREE LITERATURE Please Write to···
Dr. JOHN W. TINTERA MEMORIAL GROUP
*A.M.R.S.-Hypoglycemia foundation, inc.
149 spindle rd. hicsville, n.y. 11801
* ADRENAL METABOLIC RESEARCH SOCIETY

Judging by this notice, it is a rare person indeed who
doesn't suffer from *some* symptom of low blood sugar.

Chapter 21

The vitamin E cure-all

THE OVERPROMOTION OF VITAMINS is by now a familiar story, but in recent years one vitamin in particular has been selected by its proponents to be the savior of humanity. Vitamin E is widely promoted as a preventive, a treatment, or a cure for literally scores of human ailments — ranging from diabetes and heart disease to infertility, ulcers, and warts. It is even touted as an antidote for air pollution.

Millions of patients, it is alleged, are currently suffering from painful, crippling, life-threatening diseases because their misguided physicians refuse to recommend vitamin E supplements to them. And we are said to be rearing a new generation of children destined in turn to suffer and to die prematurely because they are not receiving daily preventive doses of vitamin E. Such claims as these have appeared in magazine articles, and in widely circulated paperback books bearing such titles as *Vitamin E for Ailing and Healthy Hearts*, *Vitamin E: Your Key to a Healthy Heart*, and *Vitamin E: Key to Sexual Satisfaction*.

Are any of these allegations justified? What is vitamin E really good for?

It was more than fifty years ago that scientists isolated a group of six or more substances called tocopherols (designated as alpha, beta, gamma, and so on). The alpha form of tocopherol was found to be the most biologically potent. In 1938 tocopherol was synthesized. However, although early research had shown alpha-tocopherol — now called vitamin E — to be a dietary essential for many animal species, no human disorder could be found for which vitamin E offered benefits. For years it remained "a vitamin in search of a disease." In 1953 Dr. M. K. Horwitt, head of the Biochemical Research Laboratory at Elgin State Hospital in Elgin, Illinois, made the first study of what happens when humans are maintained for protracted periods on low-E diets. The project spanned more than eight years — making it one of the longest as well as one of the most thorough studies of human metabolism under controlled conditions. A total of thirty-eight subjects participated in the study.

The outcome of the project can be simply stated: *There was no apparent physical or mental impairment caused by the restricted intake of vitamin E.* Low-E patients remained in satisfactory health, despite the lowering of alpha-tocopherol in their blood by 80 percent. Their red blood cells had somewhat shorter survival times — on the average, about 110 days instead of 123 — than those of the two comparison groups (those on a low-E diet who received vitamin E supplements, and those on a standard diet). But the cells remained adequate for their function. Nevertheless, the shorter survival time was considered sufficient reason for terminating the experiment. In earlier studies, monkeys maintained on diets severely deficient in vitaman E had developed anemia, and Dr. Horwitt did not want to risk that possibility with the Elgin patients. In short, the study showed that humans apparently need *some* vitamin E, but that the requirement is a modest one and can be satisfied by typical, everyday diets.

Nine patients in the project developed peptic ulcers, which showed up in X-ray examinations although not in patient symptoms. After an extensive study, experts in peptic ulcer disease concluded that the ailment was caused by factors other than vitamin E deficiency. Significantly, the incidence of ulcers was no higher among low-E patients than among those who received the same diet plus vitamin E supplements. The ulcers healed with standard therapy without complications. (Despite this experience, vitamin E is still being touted as a treatment for ulcers.)

In 1973 the National Research Council (NRC) announced a new much lower recommended daily allowance of vitamin E. The former figure for adults of 25 to 30 international units (IU) was cut by half to 12 to 15 IU (equivalent to approximately 8 to 10 milligrams of natural vitamin E in foods).

Vitamin E enthusiasts point out that millions of Americans whose intake of polyunsaturated fats is low obtain less than that amount in their diets. The deficit, they insist, should be made up by vitamin E supplements.

The fact is, however, as the NRC made clear in a June 1973 statement, that vitamin E is available in adequate quantities in the ordinary diet: "Dietary vitamin E is supplied in substantial amounts by most vegetable oils as well as by margarine and shortening made from these oils, and significant inputs are made by many vegetables and by whole-grain cereals. Meats, fish, poultry, milk, eggs, legumes, fruits, and nuts also contribute to the dietary supply."

Margarine has at least thirteen times more vitamin E than butter. A salmon steak contains ten times the vitamin E of a beefsteak, pound for pound. And most vegetable oils, which are relatively high in polyunsaturated fats, are also adequate sources of vitamin E, despite refining procedures used in processing. In short, when we eat more polyunsaturated fats, our intake of vitamin E is concomitantly increased. Even though there is an increased requirement for vitamin E in a diet high in polyunsaturated fats, that requirement is automatically met. In contrast, when the intake of polyunsaturated fats is low, the need for vitamin E is also low. "The apparent absence of vitamin E deficiency in the general population suggests that the amount of vitamin E in foods is adequate," the NRC has stated.

Vitamin E enthusiasts sometimes allege that, while ordinary diets may be good enough for ordinary good health, vitamin E supplements may lead to even better health — with greater physical vigor, strength, and endurance.

Three researchers in Britain, Drs. I. M. Sharman, M. G. Down, and R. N. Sen, subjected that possibility to a test. Thirteen boys in a boarding school swimming club were given 400 milligrams of vitamin E daily during a six-week program of intensive physical training. Before and after the six-week period, they were subjected to a variety of tests — including pull-ups, push-ups, sit-ups, breathholding, running, and swimming endurance. Significant improvement was shown at the end of the six weeks — which might lead some vitamin E enthusiasts to call out "Aha!" But thirteen other boys, matched to the thirteen test subjects in age, weight, and other criteria, were put through the same training program and evaluation. They were given a placebo similar in appearance to the vitamin E capsule taken by the test subjects. And guess what? The placebo group also improved! "No significant differences were found between the group given vitamin E and that given placebo tablets," the British researchers reported.

In addition to the claims made for alpha-tocopherol as a *vitamin*, the same chemical has for more than a quarter of a century also been touted, when used in far larger amounts, as a *medicine*. The doses specified in medicinal use commonly range from 300 to 600 milligrams a day or even higher — from thirty to seventy-five times the recommended daily allowance of the NRC.

The news magazine *Time* first broke the story of vitamin E as a medicine in its issue of June 10, 1946:

"Out of Canada last week came news of a startling scientific discovery: a treatment for heart disease (the nation's No. 1 killer) which so far has succeeded against all common forms of the ailment. . . . Large, concentrated doses of vitamin E . . . benefited four types of heart ailment (95 per cent of the total): arteriosclerotic, hypertensive, rheumatic, old and new coronary heart disease. The vitamin helps a failing heart. It eliminates anginal pain. It is non-toxic."

The clinical trials that *Time* thus enthusiastically recounted were conducted by three Canadian physicians — Dr. Evan Shute, a fellow of the American College of Obstetricians and Gynecologists and of the Royal College of Surgeons (Canada); his brother, Dr. Wilfrid E. Shute, a specialist in heart disease; and Dr. Albert Vogelsang. They based their enthusiasm for vitamin E on their personal experiences with patients. An example, reported by Dr. Wilfrid E. Shute, involved a fifteen-year-old boy who had suffered a second attack of acute rheumatic fever. During his first attack, the boy had been hospitalized for an extended period. The next time, however, Dr. Shute did not recommend hospitalization.

"The only treatment I used for the boy was 200 units of alpha-tocopherol daily," Dr. Shute reported. "In three days he was apparently well, and on the sixth day he walked into my office. He was able to return to normal farm activities. . . . This was the first case in all the world in which rheumatic fever had been treated with vitamin E."

Worldwide medical interest was aroused, of course, by this account. It was whetted even further in 1947 when the Canadian group reported on eighty-four patients of theirs treated with vitamin E. According to the group, all the patients had symptoms of angina pectoris — chest pain usually associated with coronary heart disease — and the majority had responded positively to vitamin E treatment.

Despite such glowing accounts of vitamin E benefits, the vast majority of physicians today reject vitamin E as a treatment for heart disease (and for other ailments as well). The charge is repeatedly made that the medical profession turned thumbs down on vitamin E without even trying it out. This is simply false. Vitamin E was in fact tried out — and found wanting.

By 1950 thirteen studies had been published in medical journals, all reporting the worthlessness of vitamin E during clinical trials with patients who suffered from heart disease. These reports were written by thirty-two researchers, including eminent cardiologists and professors of internal medicine. They involved more than 450 patients — as compared with the eighty-four patients on whom Drs. Shute, Shute, and Vogelsang based their initial reports.

If any of those thirteen studies had verified the claims made in Canada, further trials of Vitamin E would unquestionably have followed. News of a potential cure for heart disease compels medical attention, and no doctor or scientist could have ignored valid evidence in support of vitamin E. "We had indeed intended expanding our studies," a research group at Jewish Hospital in Philadelphia noted, "but the discouraging results presented in the preliminary report deterred us from carrying these investigations further."

Those sentiments were unmistakably representative of the medical community at large, as Dr. Herbert Eichert of Miami, Florida, confirmed during his studies of vitamin E and heart disease in 1948. In an attempt to determine the views of many heart specialists — including those who had not published any findings — Dr. Eichert sent questionnaires to department heads at medical schools throughout the United States. "Most of the clinicians," he reported, "abandoned their trials because of the utter lack of response during the preliminary phases of their investigations."

Then, in just one sentence, Dr. Eichert summed up all the medical evidence he had gathered on vitamin E's performance:

"With the exception of the claims made by Shute and Vogelsang and their group, every published, written, or verbal report which this essayist has been able to obtain indicates that vitamin E has no value in the treatment of heart disease."

In the history of vitamin E research, only a handful of field trials have complied with the rigorous standards required in compiling scientific data — and most of those trials ended with negative conclusions. The claims made for vitamin E by Drs. Shute, Shute, and Vogelsang were not based on double-blind or even on simple blind trials. Indeed CU has seen no evidence that they were even based on trials comparing patients with controls. They are essentially the uncontrolled personal impressions of three physicians who have faith in their remedy and transmit that faith to their patients. Their claims, in short, have no scientific validity.

When vitamin E is tested by physicians who are *not* enthusiasts, however, the list of failures is long. Clinical trials have failed to show any vitamin E benefits for miscarriages, sterility, menopausal disturbances, muscular dystrophies, cystic fibrosis, blood disorders, leg ulcers, diabetes, and a variety of heart and vascular diseases. The June 1973 statement by the NRC was also negative about the supposed value of vitamin E supplements for the wide variety of ailments for which vitamin E is claimed to be of benefit.

A few studies suggest that vitamin E might be useful in the treatment of intermittent claudication — a vascular condition in which the blood flow to the lower limbs is reduced and pain, most often in the calves, is experienced during walking. However, the evidence for any such benefit from vitamin E is far from conclusive, in the judgment of CU's medical consultants who reviewed the studies. The *only* therapeutic use for vitamin E in humans established by a well-controlled clinical trial is one involving the treatment of an uncommon type of hemolytic anemia in certain premature babies. Beyond that, some doctors prescribe vitamin E simply as a precautionary measure in a few relatively rare diseases involving impairment of fat absorption. Vitamin E's value in a high-oxygen environment may possibly have validity but is still not established.

The efficacy of vitamin E in toilet soaps or cosmetics for skin care, despite advertised claims, has not been scientifically established. Its possible advantage in a deodorant was ruled out when the distribution of *Mennen E* was halted by its manufacturer as a result of a rash of skin complaints from unhappy users (see Chapter 16).

CU's medical consultants believe that research on vitamin E should continue, with the aim of better defining its role in human metabolism both in healthy people and in ill people. One double-blind pilot study from Canada on the use of vitamin E in treating angina pectoris was published in February 1974. The results showed no statistically significant benefits from the use of vitamin E; however, the researcher called for a larger study of vitamin E's potential in treating cardiovascular disease.

Meanwhile, CU's medical consultants discourage, as a waste of money, the use of vitamin E as a dietary supplement or as a medication for common ailments. More important, such self-medication could lead to postponing proper medical treatment. And the cost of that could be incalculable. For now, CU's medical consultants conclude, there is no convincing evidence that human beings need more vitamin E than they obtain in their ordinary diets, or that vitamin E is useful in the treatment of any but a few rare diseases.

Chapter 22

Weight loss: diets, drugs, and devices

THE EPIDEMIC OF OBESITY spreading throughout the United States has been acknowledged by many scientists to be linked in some way to a number of other diseases, including certain forms of heart disease, diabetes mellitus, and a type of pulmonary disorder. Weight is not in itself a primary risk factor in coronary heart disease – as are cholesterol, smoking, blood pressure, and heredity, among others. However, obesity in combination with one of these primary risk factors substantially increases the chance of heart attack. There is a relationship between obesity and diabetes. The severity of the diabetes can often be reduced and the need for medication decreased by weight loss. At least one form of pulmonary disease is known to be caused by excessive overweight. And obesity can be associated with varicose veins and back troubles.

For many obese people, these potential medical complications provide more compelling reasons for weight reduction than the physical discomfort or psychological burden of massive overweight. Yet most overweight people have discovered that weight loss – and maintenance of weight loss – is no easy matter. The failure of standard low-calorie diets to diminish the problem of obesity in any permanent way has encouraged a profusion of fad diets, appetite-suppressant drugs, and reducing gadgets. However, many Americans have slenderized only their bank accounts in their quest for weight loss. Such routes to weight loss have usually proved to be dead ends. Moreover, they have sometimes introduced complications of their own.

It was only fairly recently that medical researchers began to provide some clues to the reasons why so many people tend to be overweight. In the mid-1960s, pioneering efforts by Dr. Jules Hirsch and his colleagues at the Rockefeller Institute for Medical Research (now Rockefeller University) in New York City led to the first breakthrough in understanding the nature of obesity. By means of a special biopsy and staining technique Dr. Hirsch and his co-workers were able to show that the fat patient not only had extralarge fat cells, but also an increased number of these fat cells. As patients lost weight on a low-calorie diet, the *size* of each fat cell decreased, but the *number* of fat cells remained the same. And when patients returned to previous weight levels, the size of each fat cell resumed its previous dimension.

The researchers established that the number of fat cells in each individual remains constant from about puberty onward. Using experimental animals, the study group determined the number of fat cells during the first weeks to months after birth. That number was destined to remain fairly constant for the life of the animal. Thus an animal that was relatively deprived of nourishment at that critical time of life tended to be a thinner mature animal than its well-fed littermate. It is believed likely that these observations in animals apply to human beings as well.

The plump child, whose rounded cheeks traditionally symbolized good health, may be the precursor of the obese adult. Many pediatricians, alert to current thinking about origins of obesity, make a serious attempt to limit the caloric intake of young patients. Decreasing the calories consumed in childhood may prevent a disproportionate increase in the number of fat cells, and thus possibly spare the child the plight of having to cope with the problem of obesity in the years of adult life.

Environmental influences play an important part in the problem. Widespread advertising of calorie-rich (and often nutrition-poor) foods whet the appetite. The business lunch, the testimonial dinner, the television snack, and the family get-together that makes eating the unifying activity — all can contribute to obesity.

Genetic as well as environmental factors may also be involved in the evolution of the obese adult. The child with two obese parents apparently has a greater chance of becoming obese than the youngster with only one overweight parent. And least likely to suffer from obesity is the child of two thin parents.

To some extent, economic factors are also involved. Studies have shown that among females it is the woman of means who tends to be thinner than her less affluent sister. Nor can ethnic or national origin be ruled out as contributors to obesity. Certain people, notably those of Italian and Jewish origin, tend to be more obese than those of Anglo-Saxon background.

Research into the origin and nature of obesity is still in the beginning stages. The causes of obesity are so subtle that they still defy full description. Two thousand calories a day may put weight on one individual and not on another, even though the two have the same body build and seem to engage in similar activities. So no printed chart can be relied on to tell you how many calories a day are right for you. It is not difficult, however, to determine one's proper food intake. Under ordinary circumstances, an adult whose weight is about right should eat the amount that permits maintaining this weight with little or no gain or loss. If weight begins to rise or is too high to begin with, it is time to cut down on total calorie intake. The whole problem of weight control is as simple — or as difficult — as that.

Overeating has many causes. The overwhelming majority of Americans now sit at work or at school, but national food habits stem largely from days when hard physical labor was common. A heavily laden table, in those days a necessity, is now about as useful as a buggy whip. Glandular disorders, often blamed for gross overweight, are actually quite rare. Hypothyroidism, one of the more common endocrine diseases, is the true cause of obesity in only a tiny fraction of the overweight population.

Stomach contractions leading to hunger sensations are unconditioned, primitive reflexes related to the preservation of life. The satisfaction of hunger does not lead to overeating — or to overweight. Appetite, however, is a complex, conditioned drive having both physiological and psychological components. Appetite is based on learning, on the memory of disappearance of hunger sensations and of their replacement by the pleasurable sensations of satiety, well-being, and relaxation. Appetite is also related to the agreeable taste, smell, and appearance of food. It is appetite that induces people who have satisfied their hunger with meat, bread, and vegetables to eat an appealing dessert. And in order to bring down food intake, it is appetite rather than hunger that must be curbed.

Some of those who are most concerned about weight reduction might be better off accepting their present weight level. It is certainly best to keep the weight at or slightly below the ideal for one's size, age, sex, and body build, but CU's medical consultants believe that those who are no more than about 15 percent overweight are better off doing nothing than going on and off reducing diets.

It is true that some reducing aids can bring about temporary reduction in weight, probably in large part because their use helps to put the overweight individual in the proper frame of mind to cut down on intake of food. Unfortunately, it is long-term, not short-term, weight reduction that counts, and the key to that is medically supervised dieting and exercise over a period of months or years. Even such controlled treatment fails much of the time, because obesity so often stems from emo-

211

tional and personality problems associated with eating patterns acquired over a lifetime and which are not easily changed. It is extremely rare that a shortcut approach to weight reduction brings about permanent weight control.

FAD DIETS. The appetite of many overweight Americans for the array of books touting foolproof plans for easy weight loss apparently cannot be easily curbed — even though the benefits seem to accrue primarily to the authors, publishers, and booksellers. The readers of such books can sometimes be deprived of more than their money, since some of the fad diets may endanger their health.

The 1973 commercial success in this field was *Dr. Atkins' Diet Revolution* which prescribed a low-carbohydrate regimen. The Medical Society of the County of New York called the diet "unscientific" and "potentially dangerous" — an evaluation confirmed by *The Medical Letter*, which concluded that "Although it may be effective in some patients, the Atkins diet is unbalanced, unsound, and unsafe." The aim of the diet is to produce ketosis, a condition in which body fats are burned incompletely, resulting in the appearance of so-called ketone bodies in the blood and subsequently in the urine (where they can be noted by a simple test). *The Medical Letter* points out that most diets promoting ketosis "are likely to produce fatigue, dehydration and, in some instances, nausea and vomiting, especially in persons who attempt to remain physically active." Such diets can also provoke attacks of gout and, in some people, heart irregularities. Pregnant women, especially, are warned to avoid this dietary regimen (see page 238).

"Revolution" was probably not an accurate descriptive title for Dr. Atkins' diet. The familiar *Drinking Man's Diet*, published in 1964, was also based on a low-carbohydrate scheme — with added attractions, of course. And before that, another low-carbohydrate entry was the diet advocated by Dr. Herman Taller, in *Calories Don't Count*, published in 1961. It sold well over a million copies, and many of the copies no doubt were bought by those who interpreted the title to mean that the dieters could eat all the food they wanted. These buyers were disappointed. Dr. Taller advocated a high-fat, low-carbohydrate diet, excluding not only sweets and starches but also most fruits and vegetables. The "right kind of fat," Dr. Taller claimed, "was vitally important"; polyunsaturated fatty acids supposedly "soften" body fat so that it can melt away easily.

But Dr. Taller gave no evidence that his diet was effective, beyond an account of his own experience and the experiences of some patients; he claimed there were *no* failures — highly suspect for any regimen. The one medical paper he published based on his own work, a report on ninety-three patients, showed that his tests were not controlled.

Over the years, many "new and revolutionary" diets have been promoted to the unwary — the milk diet, the milk and banana diet, the milk and corn-oil drink, the high-fat diet, the high-protein diet, and other variations and formulations variously called the Hollywood diet, the Du Pont diet, the Rockefeller diet, the seven-day, nine-day, or twelve-day diet, the *Good Housekeeping* or *McCall's* diet, and on and on. All these diets have had passing popularity. In most cases, any weight loss from such diets has been about as fleeting as their fame.

FORMULA DIET PRODUCTS. A more lasting impact on do-it-yourself reducing began when the *Metrecal* 900-calorie formula diet food was introduced about ten years ago by way of drugstores and advertisements in medical journals. Several other brands followed, and the products sold well. Such "total-diet" products are now standard items on supermarket shelves. The original powders (to be mixed with water as needed) have been largely replaced by ready-to-use liquids in cans, or by envelopes of powder to be stirred into milk. And the product lines have grown, with the addition of a variety of cookies, wafers, and soups.

Some outright cheating and false labeling by makers of these products have been detected, although the number of offenders is not large. The Food and Drug Administration (FDA) has seized powdered diets that have had less protein and more fat than declared on the label, or that have made other false nutritional claims. Most of the formula diets, however, seem to be in fact what they purport to be and are careful about claims, although it is still possible for dieters to get themselves into trouble unless they know how to use such formula diets safely (see below).

Examination of the formula of *Slender*, a strong seller among the "instant-skinny" products, discloses that it is made from skim milk, sucrose, sodium caseinate, vegetable oil, various stabilizing chemicals, and an assortment of vitamins and minerals. Four cans of ready-to-drink *Slender*, recommended for stringent dieters as a daily substitute for all other food, contain 65 grams of protein, 20 grams of fat, and 115 grams of carbohydrate, the total yielding 900 calories. The protein content may be considered adequate for a normal, healthy adult, since the suggested daily regimen provides the 65 grams of protein recommended by the National Research Council, and provides it from sources that furnish all essential amino acids. While many diet innovations involve juggling the proportions of components of the normal diet, or exclusive dependence on one or two components, *Slender*, *Metrecal*, and most competing products attempt to duplicate a well-balanced diet. They also offer simplicity and convenience of preparation. Controlled studies on the efficacy of this procedure for weight reduction are not numerous. However, almost anyone restricting intake to 900 calories daily can expect to lose weight, even without exercise.

In 1958 Drs. Alvan Feinstein, Vincent Dole, and Irving Schwartz, of the Rockefeller Institute and New York University College of Medicine, reported their observations on the use of a diet made from evaporated milk, corn oil, and sugar — the precursor of the formula now being used by *Metrecal*, *Slender*, and most similar products. Some indication of the general effectiveness of formula diets in achieving long-term weight reduction may be gained from the Feinstein group's results. They found that about 59 percent of 106 patients lost more than 20 pounds over about four months, and that about 31 percent lost more than 40 pounds. (The average starting weight was 224 pounds.) Among the advantages of the formula diets cited by Dr. Feinstein were their simplicity and inflexibility. Among the disadvantages, even for short-term use, were the monotony of the formula, gastrointestinal side effects (gas, diarrhea, or constipation) and, rarely, emotional disturbances sufficiently severe to warrant referral to a psychiatrist.

There is one other potential disadvantage of a formula diet, especially if it is used as the sole food for a prolonged period. Any attempt to reproduce a balanced diet by synthetic means runs the risk of inadvertently omitting essential nutrients usually supplied in abundance in regular meals.

In commenting on formula diets as a group, Dr. Feinstein stated that "despite the drastic nature of these substitution diets, some of the results have been dramatically good" for some patients during the relatively short periods of one to four or more months over which most such formulas have been studied. He added that the trouble with substitution diets and other special methods of reducing is that they give "falsely high results for patients who diet only briefly, and [the usual limited clinical trial] fails to indicate how close the patient has come to his [ultimate] goal" — the long-term maintenance of a reduced weight.

"Whenever complete results have been given for dietary programs," Dr. Feinstein concludes, "the data have shown that more patients fail than succeed. . . . The problem is not a lack of suitable diets or dietary adjuncts but the patient's inability to adhere to the prescribed program. . . . Consideration of all the involved factors has shown that the actual structure of the diet is of little importance as long as the patient and physician are comfortable with it."

No one should go on any diet as restricted as 900 calories without first consulting a physician. There is no harm in starting a weight reduction program with a formula diet, provided its limitations and costs are borne in mind. Dieters so inclined can cut the cost by mixing their own formula. A substitute for commercial 900-calorie diets can be made by combining, in an electric blender, about seven ounces of nonfat powdered skim milk (a little more than the amount recommended for making two quarts of milk), about two-thirds ounce of corn oil, and a quart or somewhat less of water. Sweetened with saccharin and flavored to taste with coffee or some other flavoring agent, this homemade mix is reasonably palatable. Supplemented with a vitamin/mineral capsule recommended by your physician, it is as nutritious as the commercial products but will cost you less.

It may be more convenient to use a formula diet than to choose and prepare a diet of standard foods low in calories and balanced with respect to proteins, vitamins, and minerals. Few people, however, enjoy living exclusively on a formula diet for more than a few weeks. CU's medical consultants believe that, in the long run, the use of carefully selected standard foods, combined with regular exercise, is superior to any particular formula diet product.

BEFORE-MEAL CANDIES. Typical of various dietary aids that are supposed to suppress appetite, and so help to control weight, are special candy caramels sold under a number of different trade names (*Ayds* is one of the best-known brands). The theory behind these products is that, if the level of sugar in the blood is raised just before meals, the appetite will diminish and the dieter will have no trouble at all giving up rich sauces and gravies, or declining desserts.

One leading brand, the last time CU checked, yielded about 25 calories per caramel. The directions advised that two candies be taken before meals. This is equivalent in calories to about three teaspoonfuls of sugar, an amount that actually has little effect on the blood sugar level. There is no evidence that before-meal candies suppress appetite.

Remember that when any reducing aid (candy or other) is promoted for use with a stated diet-and-exercise plan, any weight reduction achieved will more than likely be the result of the diet and exercise rather than of the reducing product.

Reducing confections often contain vitamin and mineral supplements. A moderate weight-reducing diet as low as 1,200 calories per day can be well balanced with respect to proteins, vitamins, and minerals; it can include green and yellow vegetables, skim milk or cottage cheese, eggs, lean meat, fish, fowl, fruits, and even some bread and cereals. Excluding excessive high-calorie foods does not in some mysterious way create a need for extra vitamins and minerals.

BULK PRODUCERS. Bulk-producing products swell when they absorb water. Taken about ten to thirty minutes before meals, they are supposed to swell up in the stomach and diminish hunger contractions.

Typical of the bulk producers is the vegetable product known as methylcellulose. Originally promoted for treatment of constipation (see Chapter 8), it is now sold to reduce appetite either alone or in combination with appetite-suppressing central nervous system stimulants (see below). Dieters should be warned that these products, if taken in larger than recommended doses, can have a laxative effect.

Methylcellulose and similar bulk products tend to pass fairly rapidly into the small intestine, especially when taken on an empty stomach. Even while they are in the stomach, there is no clear evidence that their presence really reduces the stomach's hunger contractions. And even if hunger contractions were diminished, this would have no bearing on the exaggerated appetite that is the major cause of overeating in obesity.

APPETITE-SUPPRESSING DRUGS. Until 1971 the most important group of appetite-suppressing agents, from the standpoint of sales, were sympathomimetic amines, drugs that stimulate the central nervous system. In 1971 slightly more than twenty-six million prescriptions (new and refills) were filled for these drugs, which have the property of affecting appetite through their action on the higher centers in the brain. Because of their widespread misuse as stimulant drugs, however, the amphetamines (Benzedrine, Dexedrine) and methamphetamines (Desoxyn, Syndrox) were reclassified in 1971 to come under the provisions of the Drug Abuse Prevention and Control Act. Under these controls, which caused an 82 percent cutback in production quotas, prescription of these drugs for use in weight reduction fell off sharply, but they were replaced in part by substitute drugs — all chemically and pharmacologically related to the amphetamines, according to the FDA.

A panel of medical consultants advised the FDA in October 1972 that the value of amphetamine-related diet drugs was "clinically trivial" and, in view of their potential for misuse, such drugs should be brought under tighter controls. The FDA proceeded along several fronts. Stricter labeling was required for these drugs to point up the limitations on their usefulness, as well as the possibility of psychological dependence. A second cut in the production of amphetamines was authorized, resulting in a total reduction of 92 percent since 1971. Amphetamines and closely related substances in injectable form were banned altogether as unsafe because of high drug abuse potential.

At the same time, amphetamines in combination with other drugs (mostly tranquilizers and sedatives) were also banned. The FDA estimated that 72 percent of the drugs prescribed by physicians as appetite suppressants were combinations of amphetamines and other drugs. Yet an FDA review of drug studies submitted by pharmaceutical firms showed that the combinations were no more effective than amphetamines used alone.

All amphetamine-type drugs prescribed as diet pills were brought under control of the Justice Department's Drug Enforcement Administration in 1973. The action imposed limitations on sales of amphetamine substitutes, but did not place them in the same highly restricted category as the amphetamines.

None of these actions affected over-the-counter (OTC) preparations for dieters. These products are being evaluated as part of the general review of all nonprescription medications now being conducted by the FDA. A drug with some pharmacological relationship to amphetamine, phenylpropanolamine, is used in OTC preparations (*Diet-Trim, Hungrex, Slender-X*) which can be bought at the corner drugstore. Interestingly enough, the same drug is used as a nasal decongestant in several cold preparations (see Chapter 2). In discussing phenylpropanolamine and its weight reduction role, *AMA Drug Evaluations* states: "This agent is probably ineffective in the dose provided (25 mg)."

There is no doubt that amphetamine drugs and related prescription medications can be used to suppress the appetite temporarily. But an effective dose varies with different individuals, and side effects are common (see below). Tolerance to these drugs is easily acquired, and after a period of several weeks increased doses may be required for continued appetite suppression.

In one careful five-year study, it was shown that excellent results in weight reduction usually were obtained in the first month or two of treatment under a physician's guidance, whether or not drugs were employed, and regardless of type. Results in patients treated by diet alone compared favorably with results in patients treated with a combination of diet and amphetamine drugs. The outcome undoubtedly reflected, in both groups of patients, enthusiasm and willingness. The study also showed side effects — dry mouth, irritability, restlessness, insomnia, rapid heartbeat, lightheadedness — from the use of amphetamine drugs.

Although studies have shown some effectiveness of appetite suppressants in the initial period of dieting (four to six weeks), the advantage over dieting managed without any drugs is so small and lasts for so short a time, and the risks of dependency are so large, that most overweight people should be advised to begin their campaign without the aid of drugs. Even the limited success possible with diet pills can come at some risk to the drug user. In addition to the side effects mentioned above, the patient may experience a letdown feeling when the drugs are no longer taken. While the effectiveness of drugs in weight reduction falls off sharply with continued usage, the same cannot be said of the possibility of dependence. A dieter may often wind up a fat person who takes amphetamines after starting out simply a fat person.

A survey of 480 physicians, published in the *Journal of the American Medical Association* in July 1973, revealed that of the doctors questioned only one-third did not prescribe appetite suppressants. And of the two-thirds who did use these drugs, most appeared to be "selective in their choice and use of drugs." However, some authorities believe that prescription of these drugs is never justified. At Senate hearings in December 1972 it was asserted that pharmaceutical manufacturers find fat people very interesting "mainly because there are so many of them." Other witnesses remarked that the pills gave doctors an easy out in dealing with their many obese patients.

PREPARATIONS CONTAINING TOPICAL ANESTHETICS. Currently in vogue are a number of OTC preparations that combine the bulk producer, methylcellulose, with benzocaine, a local anesthetic used widely in sunburn preparations and first-aid products. Currently marketed preparations containing benzocaine are: *Dexule, Pondosan, Reducets, Slim-Mint,* and *Way-Dex. Diet-Trim* offers variety — phenylpropanolamine (see page 219) is added to the usual formulation. The "rationale" behind the benzocaine-based tablet, capsule, or chewing gum is the theoretical anesthetic effect on either the lining of the mouth or of the stomach, which — allegedly — suppresses the appetite. Despite the fact that there are no controlled studies to support this contention, optimistic dieters continue to buy the idea — and the product.

EXERCISE AND MACHINES. The battle of the bulge has been joined from yet another direction, with mechanical and electrical devices for use either at home or in slenderizing salons, gymnasiums, or health clubs. Various devices may provide active exercise, passive exercise, vibration, or massage. Although these devices and the methods of using them differ, there is generally one common feature: They are promoted primarily in terms of girth reduction, as distinguished from weight reduction.

The direct value of exercise in weight reduction is easy to overestimate. But it does have a place in a well-rounded reducing program based primarily on diet. For purposes of dieting, active exercise can be defined most helpfully in terms of calorie expenditure — the number of calories used up in a given amount of time by means of a particular form of exercise (see table on page 226). After a study of the relationship between physical activity and human obesity, Drs. Anna-Marie Chirico and Albert Stunkard concluded, "The physical activity of so many obese women is so severely limited that even small increases might favorably alter caloric balance. Treatment of these women, then, might profitably encourage efforts at increasing their physical activity."

To this limited extent, then, there may be merit in appeals to the overweight by some exercise centers, so far as the claims concern swimming or other physical activities, and even in regard to machinery (at the centers or elsewhere) with which a person uses various muscles to work against weights or springs. The value of exercise in losing weight is not one of spot reducing, even when certain muscles are emphasized. It is a matter of expending calories which the body will recover from fatty tissue according to its own natural inclinations.

These are advantages of *active* exercise in which the motions of the body and contractions of the muscles are initiated by the overweight person. However, considerably less can be expected from the passive exercise provided by devices that do the initiating for you — power-driven exercise machines, rocking tables, vibrators, and other more fanciful electrical devices. One of the latter was the *Relax-A-Cizor*, a low-voltage electrical apparatus which promised to reduce girth by electrical stimulation of the muscles.

The theory behind the *Relax-A-Cizor* was that an overweight person's muscles are soft and flabby and that stimulating them to contract by means of electrical impulses improves their tone and causes them to shrink. The claims for the *Relax-A-Cizor*, so far as it can be learned, were never subjected to carefully controlled tests. What's more, the underlying theory seems to belie the biological facts. The muscles of a fat person are not necessarily soft, but rather overlaid with fat. Further, it is an *unused* muscle that shrinks; repeated contraction of a muscle should, if anything, lead to its enlargement.

In 1970 a permanent injunction against the distribution of the *Relax-A-Cizor* was issued by a United States district court. After a trial at which the views of thirty-one medical authorities were presented, the device was declared to be dangerous to health, having the potential effect of inducing abnormal rhythms of the heart, as well as causing miscarriages and aggravating such conditions as hernia, ulcers, varicose veins, and epilepsy.

Motor-driven rowing machines or bicyclelike devices yield

the benefits of exercise in proportion to the amount of effort that goes into the movements. If you merely relax on the machine and let it pull you through the motions, it may be soothing in the way a massage is soothing, and it may contribute slightly to improved muscle tone. If you really want exercise, however, it would seem more to the point to use a machine without a motor.

Perhaps the most common devices promoted for the overweight are vibrators — everything from elaborate tables, couches, chairs, and beds to cushions, belts, and small hand-held appliances at prices ranging from a few dollars to several hundred. The vibrations of several of the larger devices produce pronounced movement. They provide passive exercise in the form of rhythmic, rocking motions. What value there is in such motions is not known, but it is incorrect to assert, as has been done, that forty-five minutes on a rocking table is equivalent to playing thirty-six holes of golf or riding 10 miles at a canter. The motion can be relaxing and soothing for many people, but it cannot, in fact, have any real effect on overweight.

In most other devices the vibrations are faster and the movements smaller. Promoters of devices often claim that their products will produce a "firmer, more graceful figure" (usually in conjunction with a diet plan), and provide "exercise without effort" and "relief of tension and fatigue." Some make broader claims — relief of pain, easing the symptoms of arthritis, and relief of menstrual cramps, backaches, headaches, and high blood pressure — for which many of them have been in trouble with the FDA, since such medical claims bring the devices under the regulations of the Food, Drug, and Cosmetic Act.

All claims that vibrators are effective in promoting weight reduction or treating disease are probably false and misleading. But some of the less definite claims may have a certain basis in fact. Although comprehensive and controlled studies of the effect of vibrators on the human body have not been made, it is reasonable to assume that the devices produce effects similar to those provided by the classic massage technique. Massage has been used since ancient times to soothe tired painful joints and muscles and to induce relaxation. Massage causes a slight increase in surface blood flow and skin temperature.

However, this is far from saying that the use of a vibrating bed, pillow, abdominal belt, or other device will "tone up" muscles and reduce girth. Nor will massage (whether done by hand, vibrator device, or the mechanical rollers that pounded the hips of the girl in the television commercial) remove fat deposits under the skin. Dr. S. W. Kalb, testifying before a congressional subcommittee in 1957, reported the results of a study he had made on the effects of massage on body girth. Six weeks of twice-weekly massage of an arm and a leg produced no significant decrease in girth when compared with the unmassaged arm and leg of the same patient. In test subjects who were simultaneously dieting, decrease in girth was approximately the same in both limbs.

In some cases the federal government has come to the aid of the gullible consumer. A hearing examiner for the U.S. Postal Service ruled in March 1972 that the firm promoting *Wonder Belt* was guilty of false advertising when it claimed that its device was capable of making obese people lose weight. The Postal Service stopped payment of postal money orders for the belt, and would-be purchasers had their letters ordering the product returned to them. Prospective buyers had been taken in by claims that *Wonder Belt* would reduce the amount of fat around the user's midsection and would cause a weight loss even without a change in daily routine or reduction in caloric intake

In recent years there has been a proliferation of wearable products promoted for weight reduction — so-called sauna shorts and belts, body wraps dipped in chemical solutions, and others. All are ineffective at best, and some are downright dangerous. Doctors have warned that body wraps can be hazardous for people suffering from diabetes or diseases of the arteries and veins of the legs.

Some studies have demonstrated that a "self-help" group can be as effective in facilitating weight loss as even the most sympathetic physician. However, no one should become involved in such a project until a medical checkup has shown that dieting is indeed necessary and that dieting would not be detrimental to health.

CU's medical consultants believe there are no shortcuts to weight reduction and to weight control. Long-term weight control, even with careful medical supervision, has been achieved by only a minority of patients. In most cases, weight loss is maintained for no more than several months at a time. The shrunken fat cells in the obese dieter tend to fill out over and over again.

Almost invariably doomed to failure in the treatment of overweight are crash diets for taking off pounds quickly. Indeed, most of the weight loss achieved in the first week or two *on any diet* is due to elimination of excess water from the tissues. In order to lose 1 pound of fat, the dieter must eliminate 3,500 calories. For example, if current daily intake totals 2,700 calories, and this daily intake is lowered by 500 calories to 2,200 calories per day, weight loss theoretically should proceed at the rate of 1 pound per week — assuming all other variables remain stable. However, it is difficult to maintain constant levels of exercise; metabolic factors differ from person to person; the amount of water retained may vary from day to day. Therefore it is not unusual for someone on a calorie-restricted diet to lose weight in a highly irregular fashion, sometimes remaining at a plateau for weeks at a time.

The dieter can speed up weight loss, if desired, by increasing calorie expenditure through exercise. That exercise is self-defeating is one of the myths perpetuated by the sedentary

Exercise and calories

The following table indicates the number of calories per minute that might be expended by an individual pursuing the activities listed. The table should not be considered an absolute guide. There are far too many variables, such as physical build, age, skill at the activity, whether there is a strong wind while running, waves while swimming, or an awkward partner while dancing. CU's medical consultants suggest that you use the table as a comparative guide to the relative benefits to expect — in terms of weight loss — should you play tennis instead of golf, or paint the house instead of dig in the garden.

The data are based on material contained in Chapter 19 of *Physiology of Exercise*, Laurence E. Morehouse and Augustus T. Miller, M.D. (Saint Louis: C. V. Mosby, 1971) and in "Human Energy Expenditure," R. Passmore and J.V.G.A. Durnin, *Physiological Reviews* 35 (1955): 801-840.

Activity	Calories per minute	Activity	Calories per minute
Walking, 2 mph	2.8	Swimming/backstroke, 1 mph	8.3
Horseback riding/walk	3.0	Gardening/digging	8.6
Bicycle riding, 5.5 mph	3.2	Chopping wood	9.0
House painting	3.5	Skiing, 3 mph	9.0
Pitching horseshoes	4.0	Swimming/sidestroke, 1 mph	9.2
Walking, 3.5 mph	4.8	Figure skating	9.5
Golf	5.0	Squash racquets	10.2
Dancing/fox-trot	5.2	Fencing	10.5
Dancing/waltz	5.7	Running, 5.7 mph	12.0
Table tennis	5.8	Running, 7.0 mph	14.5
Swimming/breaststroke, 1 mph	6.8	Running, 11.4 mph	21.7
Bicycle riding, rapid	6.9	Swimming/crawl, 2.2 mph	26.7
Dancing/rhumba	7.0	Swimming/breaststroke, 2.2 mph	30.8
Swimming/crawl, 1 mph	7.0	Swimming/backstroke, 2.2 mph	33.3
Tennis	7.1		
Skating, 9 mph	7.8		
Horseback riding/trot	8.0		

obese. It is *not* true in most cases that physical activity increases food intake. However, the table on page 226 illustrates the inefficiency of exercise in losing weight as compared to calorie restriction. For example, a vigorous squash racquets game with active play lasting thirty minutes may result in an expenditure of 300 calories. The same net calorie loss can be accomplished just by passing up a single serving of lemon meringue pie.

All the answers to the treatment of obesity are obviously not yet available. As of this writing, CU's medical consultants believe that the best results for the least cost to health and pocketbook can be obtained by long-term calorie restriction, regular and well-balanced meals, and moderate exercise. For permanent results, obese people must change their life-styles — permanently.

Chapter 23

Drugs in pregnancy

GENERATIONS OF PHYSICIANS prior to 1962 were taught in medical school the comforting myth that the placenta — the organ within the uterus through which an unborn baby receives its nourishment — was a sort of guardian angel, a St. Peter at the gates of the umbilical cord, passing needed nutrients through while holding back harmful germs and chemicals. It was long known, of course, that there were some exceptions. German measles virus, for instance, could be transmitted from the mother to the embryo within the first few months of pregnancy, causing defects in the child. But not until 1962 did many physicians pay serious attention to the possibility that other dangerous substances might be passed from mother to unborn child.

In that year the world was shocked to learn that thalidomide, a drug commonly prescribed in many countries for insomnia and nervous tension, was in fact a teratogen — a substance capable of producing malformations in a fetus. Babies born to women who took thalidomide early in pregnancy suffered from phocomelia, or "seal limbs" — so called because foreshortened arms and legs resembling the flippers of seals are the most conspicuous result.

Rather than being a barrier to the transfer of drugs from

mother to fetus, "the placenta is a sieve," said the late Dr. Virginia Apgar, vice-president for medical research of The National Foundation–March of Dimes. Dr. Apgar added, "Almost everything ingested by or injected into the mother can be expected to reach the fetus within a few minutes." Alcohol, antibiotics, aspirin, barbiturates, sulfonamides, and tranquilizers are but a few of the common, and possibly harmful, substances known to pass through the placenta. Moreover, certain drugs can be found in even greater concentration in the fetal brain, heart muscle, or other organs than in the maternal tissues. In addition, the capacity of the placenta to allow transfer of some drugs seems to increase with the duration of pregnancy.

Much of this information had long been known to the relatively small group of investigators who studied the physiology of the human fetus; but little of their knowledge filtered through to practicing physicians, or even to those responsible for setting the requirements of drug testing. It took the thalidomide disaster to secure wide clinical acceptance of the established facts of fetal physiology. Physicians today assume that, when they prescribe a drug for a pregnant woman, the drug or its breakdown products – with few known exceptions – will also circulate through her unborn baby.

When pictures of thalidomide babies first hit the front pages of newspapers, many pregnant women were dismayed and immediately discontinued whatever medication they had been taking. It may be that some pregnant women still refuse to take any drugs at all.

CU's medical consultants agree that those who are pregnant – and those who wish to become pregnant – should avoid virtually all medication *for the relief of minor symptoms*, especially during the first three months (trimester) of pregnancy. However, those who are in need of medical treatment or already under the care of a doctor should be guided by their physician.

A pregnant woman can have any disease other women have. Tuberculosis, pneumonia, infectious diseases such as syphilis and gonorrhea, heart disease, epilepsy – these are but a few of the diseases that, if left untreated during pregnancy, may affect an unborn baby. Thus CU's medical consultants stress the importance both of taking prescribed medicines and of refraining from unnecessary medication.

A diabetic is a prime example of the type of patient who needs close medical supervision during pregnancy. CU's medical consultants suggest that diabetics make arrangements for medical care as early as possible in their pregnancy. Those with milder forms of the disease may do perfectly well on a special diet, and without specific medication. Those patients who are on insulin and become pregnant usually continue to take this injectable drug, which is considered safe for use in pregnancy. Those who have been taking oral diabetes medication, however, may have to switch to insulin for the duration of their pregnancy. The safety during pregnancy of such oral medications as tolbutamide (Orinase) and acetohexamide (Dymelor) has not been established. Indeed, the long-term safety of these drugs has come under serious question by some researchers.

"Why don't they test new drugs first on pregnant laboratory animals before permitting their use by pregnant women?" This question was often asked at the height of the thalidomide tragedy, and one of the results of the tragedy has been improvements in animal test procedures.

The Food and Drug Administration (FDA) guidelines for the evaluation of new drugs for use in pregnancy, announced in 1966, were stricter and better designed than earlier FDA recommendations. The guidelines even specified that a new drug be administered to male animals to check its effect on their sperm cells and their offspring. But as more and more animal tests have been run, it has become increasingly apparent that test results on animals do not always apply to humans.

That does not mean that animal tests are worthless for human protection. They can serve to arouse suspicion and to remind physicians of the need for caution. But no drug can be considered safe during pregnancy until it has actually been administered to pregnant women under carefully controlled conditions, and until the babies born to these women have been carefully studied for a period of years to check for defects not diagnosable during infancy.

Since controlled experiments on pregnant women are quite properly frowned upon, the degree of hazard associated with the vast bulk of drugs in current use has never been adequately investigated. This is why the precautions suggested by CU's medical consultants are phrased in terms of all drugs rather than just selected groups of drugs.

Some drugs, such as diethylstilbestrol (DES) — see page 239 — are believed to prevent implantation of the fertilized ovum in the wall of the uterus, thus acting as postcoital contraceptives if their use is begun within seventy-two hours after sexual intercourse. But the possibility exists that a woman who *wants* to become pregnant may use a drug that could also have this contraceptive effect, or other as yet undiscovered effects, during the period immediately following conception.

Accordingly, CU's medical consultants recommend that a fertile woman who is sexually active think of herself as potentially pregnant if she does not use contraceptive measures — and if she would not wish to abort the pregnancy should conception occur. She should discuss with her doctor any drug that may be prescribed, and at the same time restrict her use of nonprescription drugs. In this way she would enhance the possibility of having a healthy baby, should she become pregnant.

Most fetal malformations, of course, are caused by factors other than drugs and are not easily avoided. But drug-caused malformations *are* avoidable.

The thalidomide disaster served to focus popular attention

on one kind of drug damage during pregnancy — the kind likely to follow when a drug is taken between the third and the twelfth week of pregnancy. During these crucial weeks the fetus begins to assume recognizable form; the basic structures of the brain, heart, arms, legs, eyes, glands, and other organs are laid down day by day. As a result, the malformations produced also vary, depending on the stage of fetal development at which the mother took the drug.

Recent investigations have aroused suspicions about the teratogenic potential of widely prescribed antianxiety drugs — meprobamate (Equanil, Miltown), chlordiazepoxide (Librium), and diazepam (Valium) — when taken during the early months of pregnancy. An increased incidence of birth defects were found in babies born to mothers for whom these minor tranquilizers had been prescribed. Accordingly, women who wish to become pregnant should inform their doctors so that suspect drugs are not prescribed during early fetal growth.

Examples of other drugs that may be hazardous in the early stages of pregnancy are antinausea medications, such as meclizine (Bonine) and cyclizine (Marezine). These drugs can cause fetal abnormalities in experimental animals. Although there is no evidence of harm to human beings, CU's medical consultants advise against their use by pregnant or potentially pregnant women. Other well-known medications, including anticonvulsants such as diphenylhydantoin (Dilantin), have been found to be associated with an increased frequency of congenital malformations. Anticoagulants, such as warfarin (Coumadin, Panwarfin), are under suspicion as a possible cause of facial deformities in the fetus.

All women, especially pregnant women, should be wary of metronidazole (Flagyl), a drug for treatment of a vaginal infection and sold as pills and as vaginal inserts. Studies showed it to be potentially carcinogenic in humans; other studies suggest possible genetic damage. Methotrexate, a potent medication which has been prescribed for certain types of cancer, has recently been used with a fair degree of success in treating severe cases of psoriasis. Women for whom methotrexate has been prescribed should be aware that instances of fetal malformation due to this medication have been well documented. Other anticancer drugs, including mercaptopurine (Purinethol), azathioprine (Imuran), and cyclophosphamide (Cytoxan), when taken in the first few months of pregnancy, have been associated with a high rate of miscarriage.

Vaccination against rubella (German measles) is contraindicated in pregnancy. Consumers Union's medical consultants advise women who are vaccinated against rubella to avoid becoming pregnant in the first two months following vaccination. For women in the early stages of pregnancy, administration of rubella vaccine carries a small but definite risk of fetal abnormalities. When there is no adequate proof of German measles in childhood, any adult female candidate for the vaccine should be tested first for the presence of antibodies. A sample of blood can be submitted to a laboratory; many state laboratories perform the test without cost. If the test detects the presence of rubella antibodies, the vaccine need not be administered.

Because German measles and thalidomide — the two best publicized causes of prenatal malformations — have been identified as hazards in the first trimester of pregnancy, many people have gained the impression that drugs taken during other stages of pregnancy are harmless. *Not so.* For while malformations arise mostly during the first three months of pregnancy — even before the first missed menstrual period — hazards of other kinds can occur during the later stages of pregnancy.

One authority has characterized the second trimester as "the great unknown." However, two examples can be cited of drug-induced damage during the second trimester. Certain hormones of the class known as progestational agents, formerly prescribed in an attempt to avert miscarriage, sometimes produce masculinizing effects such as enlargement of the clitoris in the female fetus. (If necessary, such variations can be surgically corrected.) Substances such as iodides — present in many cough mixtures and vitamin and mineral supplements — taken during the second or third trimester may adversely affect the thyroid of the unborn baby.

Radioactive iodine, often used in the diagnosis of thyroid disorders, is absolutely contraindicated during all stages of pregnancy because it can destroy the fetal thyroid gland. For that matter, radioactivity, including ionizing radiations such as X rays, should be avoided during all stages of pregnancy, unless a physician determines that such use warrants the possible risk of fetal damage. Occasionally, pelvimetry (assessment by means of X ray of the pregnant woman's pelvis prior to delivery) may be needed by the obstetrician. If other X rays during pregnancy are absolutely necessary, routine precautions should be enforced to minimize risk to the fetus. CU's medical consultants suggest that women who are potentially pregnant take the additional precaution, when possible, of scheduling any substantial X-ray procedures or radioactive isotope tests during the ten days following the start of menstruation.

There are special risks at the end of pregnancy too — and even immediately following delivery of the infant. Several antibiotics may pose hazards, ranging from serious to mild, to the fetus as well as to the newborn baby. Sulfonamides taken by the mother shortly before delivery may increase the possibility of a certain type of jaundice in the infant. The tetracycline class of broad-spectrum antibiotics (see Chapter 28) may cause permanent staining of the unerupted tooth buds of the fetus. However, for infections that can be combated only with antibiotics, penicillin remains safe for use in pregnancy, except, of course, for those allergic to that drug.

Central nervous system depressants, such as barbiturates or

narcotics, can slow the breathing of the newborn baby if taken by the mother in high doses during labor and delivery. Anticoagulants, such as warfarin (Athrombin-K, Coumadin, Panwarfin), can cause excessive bleeding in both mother and infant at time of birth.

To call the roll of all the drugs now known to damage, or now suspected of damaging, the fetus or newborn baby would serve no useful purpose — and might lead to a false sense of security with respect to other drugs not yet adequately studied. Before any inclusive list can be compiled, intensive surveillance of birth defects, as well as studies of how pregnant women use drugs — both over-the-counter (OTC) and prescription — are required. Indeed, there is also a theoretical possibility that some medications taken *by men* may affect genetic material in sperm, and thus influence fetal development. Unfortunately, very little research has been done on this question.

A special warning is warranted about the drugs commonly found in the home medicine cabinet. So widely used a drug as plain aspirin can at delivery interfere with the coagulation mechanism of both mother and baby (see page 24). Aspirin in high doses has also been associated in at least one study with an increase in the average length of pregnancy as well as the duration of normal labor. Some learning disabilities have been observed in offspring of mice given aspirin, although there is no evidence of this phenomenon in human beings. Phenacetin, which is included in a number of familiar analgesic products such as *Bromo Seltzer* and *Empirin Compound* (see Chapter 1), has been suggested as a cause of excessive breakdown of red blood cells in the fetus or the newborn. *No* common home remedy, such as antacid preparations (see page 92), should be assumed to be completely safe in the fetus or newborn.

Even vitamins — most of them supposedly innocuous — have been known to cause harm to the unborn child when taken in excessive doses by a pregnant woman. Vitamin C, widely publicized both as a cold treatment and as a cold preventive (see Chapter 2), may possibly cause scurvy in a newborn infant if taken in high doses by the mother during pregnancy. This is due to the fact that at labor the large supply of ascorbic acid to which the infant has become accustomed — because of maternal ingestion — is suddenly stopped. High doses of pyridoxine (vitamin B_6), taken by the mother, may be associated with withdrawal seizures in the infant. Large doses of vitamin K, if administered near the delivery date, may increase the severity of jaundice in certain infants.

The hazards of excessive amounts of vitamins A and D — which exist for everyone, not just pregnant women — led the FDA in 1973 to set limits on the amounts permitted in OTC vitamin pills: 10,000 international units for vitamin A and 400 for vitamin D. Higher amounts can be obtained by prescription. The FDA statement announcing the limitation included the comment that among the ailments in which excessive amounts of these vitamins have been implicated are mental and physical retardation.

However, there is some evidence that subclinical deficiencies of certain nutrients such as vitamin C and folic acid may produce defects in the fetus. Many obstetricians prescribe vitamins in conventional therapeutic dosages for their pregnant patients. It is important that such dosages not be exceeded.

A word of caution is also in order concerning medicated salves, ointments, nose drops, suppositories, vaginal creams and jellies, and similar products applied to the skin. Such topical medications may contain substances that can be absorbed through the skin into the bloodstream and thus affect fetal development. To indicate the nature of such hazards, the FDA issues guidelines for the labeling of medications. For example, the labeling suggested by the FDA for ointments containing cortisone and related steroids (see Chapter 27) is: "Although topical steroids have not been reported to have an adverse effect on pregnancy, the safety of their use in pregnancy has not been established. Therefore, they should not be used extensively on pregnant patients, in large amounts or for prolonged periods of time."

Possible hazards to the fetus from the illicit use of narcotics, hallucinogens, and other mood-altering drugs are discussed in detail in another CU book, *Licit and Illicit Drugs*, by Edward M. Brecher and the Editors of CONSUMER REPORTS. The socially acceptable licit drugs, caffeine, alcohol, and nicotine, are known to pass the placental barrier. Studies based on animal data have implicated caffeine as a possible cause of birth defects. A study — conducted by the University of Washington School of Medicine and published in 1973 — established a link between maternal alcoholism and birth defects. The researchers concluded that the data point to serious fetal malformations as a possible consequence of alcoholism in the mother. There are few studies on "social drinking." But recent research suggests that damage to the fetus may result from intake of even relatively modest amounts of alcohol by a pregnant woman, if continued on a regular daily basis.

Pregnant cigarette smokers, however, have had ample notice that nicotine is associated with an increased risk of fetal and infant mortality. A U.S. Public Health Service report to Congress in 1973 on health implications of smoking reviewed the available research and concluded that about 4,600 stillbirths a year in the United States could probably be attributed to smoking. The report made reference to a 1972 British study on women who smoked during pregnancy, which showed a 30 percent increased risk of stillborn children and a 26 percent higher risk of infant death within the first few days after birth. However, there is some evidence that women who are able to stop smoking by the fourth month of pregnancy cut the risk somewhat. Smokers, authorities agree, tend to produce babies with a lower average birth weight than do nonsmokers.

An article published in 1973 in the *British Medical Journal* reported the results of a study of children born to mothers who smoked more than half a pack of cigarettes a day during the second half of their pregnancies. These children, at ages seven and eleven, were found to demonstrate mild degrees of mental and physical retardation.

Adequate maternal nutrition has been shown by many researchers to be of immense importance in pregnancy. It has been accepted for many years that poor nutrition results in lowered birth weights and decreased growth rates. And larger weight gains are now recommended for pregnant women than were once thought acceptable.

These findings are especially important in light of some current diet fads (see Chapter 22). CU's medical consultants strongly discourage strenuous dieting, especially low-carbohydrate regimens, during pregnancy. These may result in ketosis (the presence of ketone bodies in the blood due to incomplete burning of body fat), which has been linked with subsequent mental retardation in children born to mothers on such diets.

It is extremely difficult to detect such abnormalities as mental retardation — or behavioral defects, especially when they are minimal — and to correlate them with ingestion of substances during pregnancy. Some substances may indeed be toxic to the fetus, and these include food additives as well as drugs.

Red 2, a widely used coloring for foods and beverages (as well as drugs and cosmetics), may also affect the fetus, particularly in the period immediately following conception. The possibility that Red 2 may be a cancer-causing agent led the FDA in February 1976 to issue a ban on its further use. Because the FDA ban did not include a recall of products already manufactured with Red 2, CU's medical consultants recommend the following: All women of childbearing age, especially those in the early stages of pregnancy, should avoid artificially colored, noncola, soft drinks — unless the label clearly indicates that the product does not contain Red 2. Saccharin is another additive that may be hazardous to pregnant women. In 1975 *The Medical Letter* warned that saccharin may accumulate in fetal tissue.

Hazards to pregnancy other than those induced by drugs or chemicals are not within the scope of this chapter. CU's medical consultants suggest one exception: a warning about toxoplasmosis. This infection, when contracted in pregnancy, may do damage to the brain and other organs of the fetus. There is evidence that the organism may be transmitted to the fetus when a pregnant woman eats undercooked meat, handles a cat, or tends to a cat's litter pan. Some authorities estimate that about one-third of all adults are immune to toxoplasmosis because of previous undetected infection.

Dietary practices, environmental pollutants, emotional stress — all of these may interact in such a way as to produce subtle abnormalities, some of which may not even be recognized until many years after birth. There is evidence that some serious abnormalities do indeed take years to develop. A recent example is the discovery of a hitherto rare type of vaginal cancer in the teenage daughters of women who took diethylstilbestrol (DES) during their pregnancies in an attempt to avert miscarriage. Special techniques are required to diagnose this uncommon form of vaginal cancer. It is undetectable by the customary Pap smear test used to diagnose cervical cancer. Any DES daughter should consult a gynecologist knowledgeable in this area. Studies of DES sons have shown nonmalignant genital abnormalities in some and impaired fertility in others.

Correlation between drug use, in its broadest sense, and possible damage to the fetus or the child requires a high degree of suspicion and vigilance on the part of practicing physicians. It also requires that they follow up on any suspected side effect or risk and report to the FDA what they believe to be an adverse drug reaction.

Many suggestions have been made by competent authorities for further reducing the risks of drugs in pregnancy. Here are five proposals CU supports:

■ INCREASED UNDERSTANDING ABOUT DRUGS IN PREGNANCY ON THE PART OF PHYSICIANS AND THEIR PATIENTS. Shortly before the thalidomide disaster, a study made in California showed an incredible number of drugs — nearly eleven thousand in all — actually prescribed by physicians to 3,072 women whose pregnancies began during the year ending March 31, 1961. Only 244 of the patients (7.9 percent) went through pregnancy without a prescription; and only 563 (18.3 percent) had only one drug prescribed; 617 women received more than five drugs each, and 121 received ten or more. A few received twenty or more different drugs. These totals did not include self-prescribed drugs, OTC drugs, or drugs prescribed before pregnancy that patients continued to take during pregnancy. And keep in mind that some prescriptions can contain more than one drug ingredient. The actual number of risks was considerably higher, because one drug alone may be effective and safe but may be rendered ineffective or harmful when taken at the same time as one or more other drugs.

Some of the drugs prescribed were no doubt essential for the health or well-being of the patient or her unborn baby; but many others were probably superfluous. For example, 426 of the 3,072 women received prescriptions for medicated lotions or creams (usually for skin conditions), 716 received analgesics, 443 were prescribed antiobesity drugs or appetite suppressants, 533 received antihistamines (mostly because they had colds), 605 received barbiturates or other sedatives and hypnotics, and so on down the long list.

How much more cautious are physicians today when they write prescriptions for their pregnant patients? No one really knows. But the evidence is not encouraging. In 1971 the *British Medical Journal* published a report that more than 97 percent of the 1,369 pregnant women included in a study took drugs prescribed by their doctors, and 65 percent of them practiced self-medication. A later survey in Scotland seemed to confirm these findings. Of the 911 women included in the Scottish study, 82 percent were prescribed drugs (exclusive of iron) during pregnancy — with an average of four drugs prescribed for each woman — and 65 percent of the pregnant women dosed themselves with OTC preparations. In the United States, a study centered in Houston (and reported to a 1973 symposium sponsored by The National Foundation–March of Dimes) revealed that each pregnant woman participating in the survey took an average of ten different drugs. One participant in the Houston study — confined to women in middle- and upperclass socioeconomic groups — who took twenty-five aspirins daily during her pregnancy reported that she would never have done so had she known aspirin was a drug.

In view of these findings, CU recommends that educational programs about drugs in pregnancy — for doctors and the general public alike — be given priority. Doctors should be strongly encouraged to consider the risks when prescribing or advising medication for a pregnant patient — or for a potentially pregnant patient. And if medication is warranted, a patient should be warned to take drugs only in prescribed amounts and for specified durations. There is urgent need for clearly worded warnings and guidelines to be prepared for distribution to pregnant women by doctors, pharmacists, clinics, and other health agencies.

■ INTERNATIONAL COOPERATION IN TESTING. Following the thalidomide disaster, the United States, Canada, Britain, France, Germany, and other countries tightened up animal test procedures. In most respects, foreign test requirements are less strict than the FDA guidelines. In some testing programs, however, there is too much costly duplication. Substantially the same test, with only minor variations, must be run over and over again to satisfy the requirements of all the countries in which a new drug is to be marketed. If the FDA and comparable agencies in other countries could agree upon a series of test protocols, money now wasted in duplicate tests could be devoted to a far broader battery of additional tests.

The FDA has now formulated guidelines under which certain clinical drug studies performed abroad would be acceptable in this country as part of the review process preliminary to approval of any new drug application. In this way research data accumulated outside the United States would not need to be duplicated as long as the studies conform to generally recognized international standards. In a proposal filed in September 1973, the FDA announced that its standards for acceptability would be based on the recommendations of the Eighteenth World Medical Assembly, which met in Helsinki, Finland, in 1964. When fully operative, the FDA program may lead the way to increased international cooperation in testing procedures.

■ PRIMATE TESTS. Most new-drug pregnancy tests are now performed on rats, mice, and rabbits. The FDA "encourages" tests on pregnant monkeys but does not require them; they are rarely run because they are so expensive. Would tests on monkeys or other primates more closely related to man than rats, mice, and rabbits secure results more valid for pregnant women? No one really knows; there have been too few primate tests. A large-scale research program designed to determine whether primate tests are worth the extra cost is thus a third recommendation.

■ IMPROVED PACKAGE INSERTS. Before any drug can be marketed, the pharmaceutical firm responsible must secure FDA approval of a "package insert" or "product information circular," which lists precautions and contraindications as well as indications, dosages, and other important data. One difficulty with package inserts as a means of alerting busy physicians to the hazards of a drug they are prescribing for a pregnant woman is purely a question of format and type size. The information about pregnancy may consist of only a few words buried in a thousand words or more of small type on other subjects. It may appear under "Precautions" or "Contraindications," or possibly somewhere else. It may even be a single word hidden in the middle of a long sentence, as in this example: "To be given with caution in the presence of diabetes mellitus, pregnancy, hypothyroidism, epilepsy, cerebral damage, chronic and acute nephritis."

How many busy physicians miss the key word printed in small type is anybody's guess. CU's proposed reform is therefore elementary: Along with the paragraphs conspicuously headed "Dosage and Administration," "Precautions," and "Contraindications," each package insert should be required to carry pregnancy warnings in a separate paragraph conspicuously headed "Usage in Pregnancy." This practice is presently followed for a number of drugs whose package inserts list information relevant to pregnancy under a clearly labeled heading of suitable type size. Occasionally, the heading reads "Usage in Pregnancy and the Child-Bearing Age" — an even more informative title. Unfortunately, in many other package inserts the information appears as an unlabeled item under "Warnings," or even "Dosage and Administration," or "Contraindications." Standardization of format would help eliminate confusion about where the physician should look for information about drug hazards in pregnancy. Uniformity in title and placement, together with a requirement for prominent type, should also be enforced by the FDA. As of this writing, the FDA is preparing to issue new regulations concerning package inserts. Some of the reforms advocated by CU may be included.

All the above suggestions about improving package inserts deal with material addressed to physicians. CU believes that patients have a right to direct access to information about the implications of drug usage. At the present time oral contraceptives (and two other contraceptive drugs) are the only prescription drugs for which manufacturers include FDA-approved package inserts prepared for the use of patients. In general, CU endorses this practice and would like to see it extended to cover other medications, starting with those likely to be hazardous during pregnancy.

■ REPORTING OF ADVERSE EFFECTS. The thalidomide hazard was unmasked when physicians in West Germany and Australia noted a sudden, startling increase in infant malformations of a type encountered only rarely before. Improved procedures for reporting events of this kind have been instituted. It is unlikely that if another drug like thalidomide comes along its teratogenic effects would be overlooked until ten thousand babies have been afflicted.

But the problem has not been solved. We can hardly expect that the next teratogen will produce such a dramatic and readily recognizable pattern of otherwise rare defects. The next new drug may produce mental retardation, for example, or premature birth or some other already common misfortune. If so, it may affect thousands of babies without revealing itself; such afflictions could easily go unnoticed among the countless similar cases already occurring. What is needed as an alerting mechanism is continuous registry of the occurrence of all malformations and other perinatal conditions in an entire population. Then, if some common condition is seen to be increasing in frequency, a search for causes can be promptly undertaken.

In 1951 the Canadian province of British Columbia developed a registry for the reporting of major birth defects; minor birth defects were also recorded beginning in 1963. Since 1970 four other provinces have joined with British Columbia in a federally coordinated surveillance program for reporting defects detected during the first year after birth. In the United States, the first comparable program was begun in 1967 and covers metropolitan Atlanta. Six Florida counties have monitored birth defects since 1971; a program for the state of Nebraska was initiated in May 1973. However, it was not until November 1974 that the large-scale registry of birth defects began in the United States. About 1,500 hospitals nationwide are participating in the new Birth Defects Monitoring Program, which is being coordinated by the Center for Disease Control in Atlanta.

Surveillance of approximately one million births yearly will be based on computer data compiled from records of the participating hospitals. Limitations are built into the monitoring system, however, since hospital records do not include such information about the newborn's mother as age, number of previous pregnancies, and medications taken during pregnancy. Although the Canadian and United States programs would undoubtedly discover any disaster on the scale of the thalidomide tragedy, these systems probably cannot detect the causes of small clusters of birth defects. Even the more sophisticated Canadian system does not provide for the kinds of information necessary to establish a clear connection between birth defects and maternal drug use.

Authorities on surveillance of birth defects believe some relatively simple changes would improve the effectiveness of monitoring programs. Procedures for linking birth defects with maternal factors could probably be strengthened if terminology were standardized, hospital records were kept in a uniform fashion, and hospital admission records for infants required information about the mother (such as her age).

We have stressed the drug factor in malformations and other problems of fetuses and newborn babies because something can be done about it right now, both by patients and by the medical profession. But it is also important to keep the drug factor in proper perspective.

The great majority of malformations and other unfortunate

outcomes of pregnancy are caused by factors other than drugs. Even those California women who received as many as twenty drugs apiece during pregnancy for the most part delivered healthy babies. However, 175 of the 1,369 mothers in the British study gave birth to infants with major congenital abnormalities during the study period. But the number involved is not the only crucial factor. Drug hazards should not be stressed because the ill effects are so numerous or so likely to occur, but because when they do occur they can in some cases be so devastating. And in most instances, the hazards of drug taking can be easily avoided. Pregnant women who follow CU's precautions, listed below, and whose physicians use ordinary prudence in prescribing for their patients, can be assured that the risks and side effects of drugs in pregnancy can be minimized.

CU's medical consultants recommend that the following cautions be observed by pregnant women, as well as by fertile women who engage in sexual intercourse without contraception and who wish to become pregnant:

▪ No chemical has been proved to be entirely harmless for all pregnant women and their unborn babies during all stages of pregnancy. Therefore, do not take any drug unless there is a specific medical need for it. Be especially careful in the first trimester of pregnancy and just before delivery.

▪ If there *is* a medical need, and if your physician prescribes a drug to meet that need, take it only in the amounts and at the times specified. Do not increase or reduce the dose; do not discontinue usage sooner or continue it longer than directed. Remember that your unborn baby's health can be adversely affected by your failure to take a needed drug, as well as by your indulgence in unprescribed medication.

▪ A number of drugs exert their adverse effects during the first weeks following a missed menstrual period – the weeks when you are likely to be wondering whether you are pregnant.

Therefore, if pregnancy is a possibility, discontinue all self-prescribed remedies within a few days after an expected menstrual period fails to occur, and recheck with your doctor concerning drugs previously prescribed for you. If you are trying to become pregnant, be sure to tell your doctor this if a drug is prescribed for you.

■ During pregnancy and also during the time you may wish to become pregnant, curtail the use of OTC "home remedies," as well as drugs available only on a doctor's prescription.* Even common self-prescribed medicines, such as aspirin, should be taken sparingly — except on your doctor's advice.

■ Interpret the term "drugs" broadly to include many things besides oral preparations and injections — for example, lotions and ointments containing hormones or other drugs that may be absorbed through the skin, and vaginal douches, suppositories, and jellies.

* Mothers who breast-feed their babies should continue to avoid the use of medications as much as possible. Numerous drugs taken by the mother are excreted in her milk and reach the nursing baby. If you are nursing your baby, be sure to report this to your family doctor should medication happen to be prescribed.

Chapter 24

Insomnia, tension, and anxiety

AT ONE TIME OR ANOTHER almost everyone experiences difficulty in falling asleep or in staying asleep. And just about everyone, in varying degrees, eventually becomes susceptible to the idea of "taking something" to assure a good night's sleep. Drugs purported to induce sleep have been available without prescription for many years now. And recently, Americans have been urged by drug manufacturers to try *daytime* sedatives as well, to relieve feelings of anxiety or tension. Several million people, drugstore sales figures show, now look to over-the-counter (OTC) medication for relief of pressures resulting from the frustrations of everyday life.

What are the facts about insomnia, and just how safe and effective are the various drugs used for it? Occasional mild difficulty in sleeping may have various causes. Tensions, aggravated by the social and economic problems that are a part of everyone's life, are often to blame. Sometimes, insomnia may be due to excessive use of caffeine beverages, such as coffee, tea, cocoa, or cola drinks. Also capable of spoiling a good night's sleep are certain prescription drugs. These include stimulants such as dextroamphetamine (Dexedrine) or methylphenidate (Ritalin), sometimes used to combat mental depression, and appetite-suppressant drugs for treatment of obesity, such as diethylpropion (Tenuate) and phenmetrazine (Preludin).

A healthy adolescent or adult usually does not suffer any harm, temporary or permanent, from occasionally missing a few hours of sleep or even an entire night's sleep. In fact, the supposed sleeplessness may be more apparent than real; you may have all the sleep your body really needs. The traditional notion that it is necessary to sleep eight hours each night has no basis in fact. Adults vary a great deal in sleep requirements, some functioning effectively with only five hours' sleep a night while others require eight or nine hours.

Infants and children, too, show marked variation in sleep habits and needs. Investigators in Rochester, Minnesota, studied the sleep habits of a group of 783 children, aged two to three. They discovered that the total number of hours slept in a twenty-four hour period ranged from eight to as much as seventeen hours; the average was thirteen hours. An occasional interruption in the usual sleep pattern of a child did not result in physical or mental harm.

There is more reason for concern over persistent, severe insomnia — difficulty either in falling asleep or in remaining asleep almost every night. This kind of insomnia is also rather common. In rare cases, it may be due to organic brain disease; more frequently, it may result from pain, breathlessness, asthma, cough, or the need for frequent urination. In these instances, successful treatment of the underlying disorder should solve the insomnia problem. Most often, however, severe or chronic insomnia is a symptom of tension, or even of a neurosis. Because psychotherapy is not always available, or because of its high cost, most anxieties and their accompanying insomnia are either self-treated or treated by the family doctor, generally with sedatives or tranquilizers.

Among the popular methods of self-treatment for persistent insomnia are: warm baths; warm milk or a hot toddy; the employment of various mechanical devices, such as special mattresses, bed lights, ear plugs, and eye shades; redecorating the bedroom; and listening to recordings of soothing, monotonous music, or of the hypnotic voice of a "psychologist" who, with lulling words, phrases, sounds, and rituals, attempts to help insomniacs control their depressed or anxious psyche. Unfortunately, none of these methods can help confirmed insomniacs. Some traditional remedies may even inhibit sleep. For example, that bedtime cup of cocoa — just like coffee and tea — contains caffeine, a stimulant drug.

For many years insomnia was treated by physicians with alcohol (a "nightcap" to induce sleep) or with sleeping potions made from either chloral hydrate (knockout drops) or paraldehyde, which were among the earliest drugs found to depress the central nervous system — the standard approach to sleep inducement. But not everyone accepted alcohol as medication; some embraced it too enthusiastically. And the drugs had an objectionable taste and smell. Thus when barbiturates — which are also central nervous system depressants — became available early in this century, the medical profession adopted them for patient care. As hypnotics (in distinction to their use as daytime sedatives), barbiturates, especially the short-acting ones, such as pentobarbital (Nembutal) and secobarbital (Seconal), are the most effective. However, regular and prolonged use of this type of barbiturate carries with it some risk of addiction. For these reasons, a physician closely supervises treatment of insomnia with barbiturates or with any similar drug (see below). The Food and Drug Administration recently placed barbiturates on the list of controlled substances in an attempt to restrict their nonmedical use* (see page 264).

*The nonmedical use of barbiturates and of other psychoactive drugs is explored in another CU special publication: *Licit and Illicit Drugs — The Consumers Union Report on Narcotics, Stimulants, Depressants, Inhalants, Hallucinogens, and Marijuana — including Caffeine, Nicotine, and Alcohol*, by Edward M. Brecher and the Editors of CONSUMER REPORTS, 1972, 623 pages.

Because of concern about the increasing nonmedical use of barbiturates, the medical profession has in recent years turned to newer varieties of central nervous system depressants. However, these prescription sedatives, such as glutethimide (Doriden), ethchlorvynol (Placidyl), and flurazepam (Dalmane), differ only slightly in pharmacological action from barbiturates, and the potential danger of dependency or addiction from such drugs is approximately the same as for barbiturates. *AMA Drug Evaluations* commented about hypnotics: "Long-term use of larger than usual therapeutic doses may result in psychic and physical dependence." Furthermore, a controlled study, reported in 1974 in the *Journal of the American Medical Association (JAMA)*, demonstrated the relative ineffectiveness of hypnotic drugs — barbiturates and other central nervous system depressants — when taken by insomniacs over a two-week period.

Another class of prescription drugs, which are normally prescribed for tension or anxiety but are sometimes taken for insomnia, are the minor tranquilizers such as meprobamate (Equanil, Miltown), chlordiazepoxide (Librium), diazepam (Valium), and others. For a discussion of their use and effectiveness, see Chapter 25.

The nonprescription sedatives and sleep aids are neither tranquilizers nor barbiturates. *Dormin, Nite Rest, Nytol, Sleep-Eze,* and *Sure-Sleep,* like almost all other OTC sleeping preparations, contain as their main sedative ingredient an antihistamine drug, usually methapyrilene (known by the trade name Histadyl). *Nytol* and *Sure-Sleep* also contain a small amount of an analgesic, salicylamide. *Nite Rest, Sleep-Eze,* and *Sure-Sleep* contain scopolamine (also called hyoscine), a mild sedative derived from belladonna. The amount of scopolamine present in most such OTC preparations is too small to have any significant sleep-inducing effect when used as directed, nor is there any evidence that it increases the effectiveness of the antihistamine in overcoming sleeplessness. However, with minimal overdosage or prolonged usage, untoward reactions to scopolamine, including possible behavioral abnormalities, may occur (see page 253).

As widely advertised as OTC products "to induce restful sleep" at night are those touted "to relieve nervous tension." The latter group includes *Compoz*, which its manufacturer claims is the "largest-selling nonprescription sedative for temporary relief of simple nervous tension." According to a study conducted by Dr. Karl Rickels of the University of Pennsylvania School of Medicine, which appeared in a January 1973 *JAMA*, this way of dealing with mild anxiety is not only rarely a help in obtaining relief of symptoms, but it may actually induce unwanted side effects, some serious in nature.

The main purpose of the Rickels study was to compare *Compoz*, aspirin, placebo, and chlordiazepoxide (Librium), a minor tranquilizer available by prescription, in terms of safety and effectiveness in decreasing nervous tension and combating anxiety. The article reported that *Compoz*, an OTC medication containing two antihistamines (methapyrilene and pyrilamine) as well as scopolamine, was no more effective than aspirin *or a placebo* in providing relief for mild-to-moderate anxiety, and that the prescription medication, chlordiazepoxide, achieved significantly better results than any of the three other methods of treatment.

But on the negative side, *Compoz* led the field. *Compoz* was highest in percentage of patients reporting side effects and in overall number of side effects reported. Furthermore, *Compoz*, when compared with chlordiazepoxide, produced a larger number of side effects rated by physicians as "marked" (eight versus one) and "moderate" (fifteen versus eleven), but fewer rated as "mild" (eight versus twelve).

Scopolamine is used in many OTC sleep aids and sedatives, including *Compoz*. Scopolamine may produce — even when medication is taken as directed — such effects as dry mouth, blurred vision, increased pressure in the eyes, and difficulty in urination. People who have closed-angle glaucoma — and a significant number do, without knowing it (see Chapter 6) — should avoid sleep remedies containing scopolamine since it may cause a further increase in pressure within the eyes. And if taken in higher doses and after prolonged usage, medications containing scopolamine can cause "mental confusion, excitement, and delirium," according to the Rickels study.

Actually, *Compoz* contains a much smaller amount of scopolamine (0.15 milligrams) when compared with many other OTC tranquilizers, which were not included in the Rickels study. The top scorer in this category is *Sominex Capsules* (0.5 milligrams); other products with scopolamine include *Nite Rest*, *San-Man*, and *Sominex Tablets* (each 0.25 milligrams); *Sure-Sleep* (0.2 milligrams); and *Seedate* and *Sleep-Eze* (each 0.125 milligrams). In fact, the ads for *Nytol* capitalize on the absence of scopolamine in its formulation, and call its "gentle combination of ingredients" (an antihistamine and an analgesic) "both effective and safe."

All the above medications also contain about 25 to 50 milligrams of methapyrilene, an antihistamine. (*Compoz* contains a second antihistamine as well.) *The Pharmacological Basis of Therapeutics*, edited by Drs. Louis S. Goodman and Alfred Gilman, lists the following among the potential side effects of antihistamines — aside from sedation: dizziness, incoordination, blurred vision, nervousness, anorexia (loss of appetite), frequent urination, skin rashes, and sometimes blood changes. These side effects, which probably are not frequent when the sleep products are used according to directions, might appear with larger doses and could persist for many hours. Such side effects as dizziness and prolonged sleepiness can, of course, be dangerous to many — a driver or one who works with a machine, for example.

How effective are nonprescription sleep aids depending on scopolamine and antihistamines? Dr. Louis Lasagna, Professor of Pharmacology and Toxicology at the University of Rochester School of Medicine and Dentistry, has written: "Presumably these [antihistamine and scopolamine] drugs have come to be promoted as hypnotics because of the drowsiness observed as a side effect attendant on their use in the treatment of allergic disorders and in the prevention of motion sickness. How effective are the preparations? No one really knows. Every physician . . . is aware of the ability of most antihistamines, given in sufficient dosage, to affect the central nervous system, sometimes with resultant stimulation, usually with sedation, occasionally with both."

In other words, they may work for some people some time. But in chronic, persistent insomnia it is unlikely that these drugs are ever consistently effective. Indeed, some people may never find them effective, no matter what type of insomnia they suffer from.

Just as important, how safe are these OTC drugs? It is probably safe enough to use them from time to time, *according to label directions*. But if you find that the small recommended doses are ineffective, it is certainly unwise to take larger doses.

One daytime product with a different approach is *Nervine*, an OTC preparation described as a "calmative" by its manufacturer. *Nervine* depends on bromides for its action. *AMA Drug Evaluations* describes bromides as "useless as hypnotics" and then concludes: "Since bromides accumulate in the body and can cause severe drug-induced psychoses, their use is deemed unadvisable." Bromides may precipitate skin rashes (see page 118), and can be toxic if used extensively. Although it is true, as *Nervine* claims, that "bromides have been used for many years in the treatment of functional nervous symptoms," the trend in recent years has been to omit bromides from OTC formulations — as is now the case with *Bromo Seltzer*. Apparently, most drug manufacturers accept the AMA verdict on bromides.

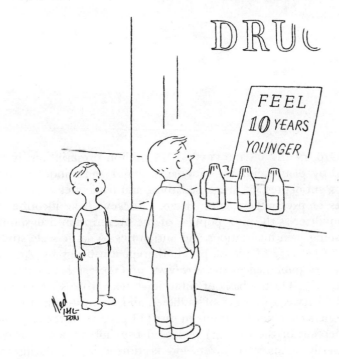

"But why would anybody *want* to feel ten years younger?"

Chapter 25

Psychotherapeutic drugs

IN 1970, IN THE UNITED STATES, 214 million prescriptions were filled by pharmacists for stimulants, major and minor tranquilizers, antidepressant drugs, sedatives, and hypnotics — the main types of psychotherapeutic drugs.* Surveys have identified a tranquilizer as the most popular of the prescription drugs, outstripping pain medications and antibiotics. A large-scale study of the patterns of use of psychotherapeutic drugs by Americans was published in the *Archives of General Psychiatry* in June 1973. On the basis of interviews with a cross section of adults between the ages of eighteen and seventy-four, the researchers concluded that one in five (13 percent of the men and 29 percent of the women) had used psychotherapeutic drugs, primarily minor tranquilizers and daytime sedatives, during the period of the survey — late 1970 and the spring of 1971. The study included the use of amphetamines, which had not yet been ruled a controlled substance (see Chapter 22).

Most users, according to the survey, felt they were helped by

* For a pioneering report on the nonmedical use of mood-altering drugs, see *Licit and Illicit Drugs — The Consumers Union Report on Narcotics, Stimulants, Depressants, Inhalants, Hallucinogens, and Marijuana — including Caffeine, Nicotine, and Alcohol,* by Edward M. Brecher and the Editors of CONSUMER REPORTS, 1972, 623 pages.

psychotherapeutic drugs; three of four reported the drugs helped them "a great deal" or "quite a bit." The data indicated that use of these prescription drugs was twice as high for women as for men, most of the difference being attributed to the more frequent use by women of drugs in the minor tranquilizer/sedative group. The study pointed out that men would surpass women as drug users if certain other mood-altering drugs — notably alcohol and marijuana — were included.

Is anything much being accomplished by the hundreds of millions of psychotherapeutic pills Americans swallow annually? The answer depends in large part on which drugs are under consideration. Three major classes of psychotherapeutic drugs are commonly prescribed by physicians: antianxiety, antidepression, and antipsychotic drugs.

Antianxiety drugs — the minor tranquilizers — are commonly prescribed for such symptoms as anxiety and nervous tension. Authorities agree that they have a calming effect similar to that of barbiturates. Some studies indicate that the minor tranquilizers, while producing their desired antianxiety response, cause less of an annoying side effect — drowsiness — than the older barbiturates. Meprobamate, sold under the trade names Equanil and Miltown, is the first of the antianxiety drugs. The table on page 278 lists others in general use today.

Antidepression drugs, also listed in the table, are not tranquilizers. As their name implies, they are prescribed for depressed patients. In general, they tend to stimulate rather than depress the central nervous system, although some of them may, in addition, have sedative or other effects.

Antipsychotic drugs — including the major tranquilizers — have proved particularly effective against schizophrenia and other psychoses, although they have other uses as well. Chlorpromazine, sold under the trade name Thorazine, was the first of these drugs; more than a dozen other antipsychotic drugs are now marketed (see table on page 278).

All three of these classes of drugs are available only by prescription. Over-the-counter (OTC) remedies that purport to be "tranquilizers" are generally mild sedatives or antihistamine drugs with mildly sedative side effects. Or the drugs may be formulated in combination — as in *Compoz*, which contains methapyrilene and pyrilamine (antihistamines) and a low dose of scopolamine (a drug with a mildly sedative effect; see page 253 for a discussion of side effects). Variations of this mixture are commonly used in daytime OTC sedatives and also in some OTC sleep-inducing products, such as *Nite Rest* and *Sleep-Eze* (see Chapter 24).

The most comprehensive studies of all three classes of psychotherapeutic drugs have come from the Department of Medicine and Surgery of the U.S. Veterans Administration (VA). Almost sixty-five thousand patients were treated in thirty-three VA psychiatric hospitals in the year ending February 1973, and many tens of thousands of additional patients rely on the VA's 136 general hospitals and 83 mental hygiene clinics for care. Thus the VA patient population includes moderately troubled patients as well as severely ill ones. Out of this wide experience and out of the VA's "Cooperative Studies of Chemotherapy in Psychiatry" have come a series of distinguished reports on the effects of psychotherapeutic drugs.

A similar series of studies has been performed by hospitals and clinics participating in "collaborative study groups" established by the Psychopharmacology Research Branch, National Institute of Mental Health (NIMH). Both the VA and the NIMH studies use many treatment centers across the country, so that the results are not distorted by favorable or unfavorable factors unique to a particular center or to the kinds of patients it attracts. The description which follows relies primarily on the VA and NIMH reports, on a chapter by Dr. Murray E. Jarvik, of the University of California at Los Angeles School of Medicine, in a leading textbook on drug therapy (*The*

Pharmacological Basis of Therapeutics, edited by Drs. Louis S. Goodman and Alfred Gilman), and on the judgments of CU's medical consultants.

ANTIANXIETY DRUGS (THE MINOR TRANQUILIZERS)

According to ads addressed to physicians in leading medical journals, these are indeed miracle drugs. One product, it was alleged, "helps restore the zest for living." Another was said to be useful "in emotional distress." A third "controls anxiety, tension, agitation, irritability, anxiety-linked depression," and so on. The ads urged physicians to prescribe one antianxiety drug for "emotional crises in office practice" and "to gain more immediate control of acute agitation and tension." Another drug was offered for the emotional aspects of physical illnesses — "when constant business worries aggravate peptic ulcer symptoms" or "when constant family pressures aggravate the symptoms of mild ulcerative colitis." Yet another drug was recommended "when your patient's worries, apprehensions, or other manifestations of acute and chronic anxiety interfere with his sleep." Then "a bedtime dosage . . . helps break the anxiety-insomnia cycle."

The ads were for the most part based on the reports of physicians who had tried antianxiety drugs in their practices. Typical of such uncontrolled studies was one reported by a physician who prescribed diazepam (Valium) for seventy-four patients — men and women who came to him complaining of inability to sleep, "nervousness," tension, fatigue, crying spells, restlessness, headache, and so on. The results seemed promising indeed. Of the seventy-four patients given diazepam, "improvement was marked in forty-five (60.8 percent), moderate in twenty (27 percent) and minimal in nine (12.2 percent)." Apparently, none failed to improve. Other uncontrolled studies of diazepam also brought glowing reports. One enthusiastic physician claimed that 58 to 93 percent of patients benefited.

In addition to such findings by physicians and their patients, there are reports from the fully controlled VA and NIMH clinical trials. In such trials, some patients are given the drug under study, while others, selected at random, are given placebos which look just like the study drug but contain no active ingredient. The controlled trials are usually double-blind — neither the patients who receive the pills nor the physicians who give them and evaluate their effects know which patients receive the study drug until after the results have been recorded. Crossover trials are also run: The patient receives the study drug for a while, then the placebo, and then the study drug again. Neither the patient nor the physician is informed when the crossover takes place. In short, effectiveness is not judged solely by the patient's belief that medication has been beneficial, or by the doctor's impressions, although these are taken into account. In many studies, objective tests are also given before and after drug or placebo treatment, and the patient is evaluated on the basis of test scores.

When antianxiety drugs are tested in these sophisticated ways, a remarkable pattern is noted. In one controlled, double-blind study, for example, half of the patients given diazepam were judged to be significantly improved after six weeks on the basis of both objective tests and the physician's judgment. *But half of the patients given a placebo were also found to be significantly improved.*

With a few exceptions, the results of fully controlled trials using other leading antianxiety medications have been much the same. "Drugs such as meprobamate (Equanil or Miltown) and chlordiazepoxide (Librium) generally come out as being a little better than a placebo, but not by any dramatic margin," reported Dr. Jonathan O. Cole, formerly in charge of NIMH drug research studies and now superintendent of Boston State Hospital.

In 1973, in the *Journal of the American Medical Associa-*

tion, Dr. Karl Rickels of the University of Pennsylvania reported the results of a study comparing the efficacy of chlordiazepoxide (Librium, a prescription drug), *Compoz* (an OTC preparation), aspirin, and a placebo. Of the four, Librium was found to be the most effective in relieving anxiety, depression, and other related symptoms (see Chapter 24).

Doubts also exist about the relative effectiveness of the minor tranquilizers as compared with that of sedatives, such as barbiturates. "It has been suggested that the gap between the antianxiety dose and the dose causing drowsiness and dizziness is greater for the newer sedative-tranquilizers than for the barbiturates," *The Medical Letter* told its readers. "But it has not been clearly established that there is such a difference." And according to Dr. Jarvik: "The pharmacological effects of meprobamate are very similar to those of barbiturates. Indeed, in clinical usage it is difficult, if not impossible, to differentiate between the two drugs."

Not all authorities agreed with this view. "Our experiences in the VA would certainly give the antianxiety drugs higher marks than the barbiturates, both as to efficacy and safety," said Dr. Samuel C. Kaim, formerly in charge of VA research in psychiatry and neurology. "In several double-blind studies, meprobamate and chlordiazepoxide have turned out to be better than either barbiturates or a placebo." This is also the view of the countless physicians who prescribe antianxiety drugs, and of the patients who report benefits from them. Although no final resolution of this controversy is in sight, *AMA Drug Evaluations* commented that antianxiety agents "may be useful for patients in whom the sedative-hypnotics cause an excessive loss of alertness."

Dr. Cole called attention to another curious point. "In a series of studies involving three out-patient clinics," he noted, ". . . we have been most struck by the fact that the results differ substantially from clinic to clinic, to the extent that if each clinic were considered as a single study, quite different results would have been reported. . . . These differences cannot be accounted for by the known characteristics of the patients treated."

The explanation may lie in this comment by Dr. Jarvik: "The reaction of the patient to meprobamate may be strongly influenced by the physician's attitude. In one study in which meprobamate, phenobarbital [a barbiturate sedative] and a placebo were administered in a double-blind fashion to patients, it was found that physicians who were enthusiastic about the possible results of drug therapy obtained better results than did those who were pessimistic or skeptical."

To sum up the evidence on effectiveness, the odds are better than fifty-fifty that a patient given an antianxiety drug by a physician will be benefited. Patients in need of sedation are the ones most likely to benefit. If the physician has faith in the drug, the results are likely to be better. These findings explain why antianxiety drugs are so popular. Whether they work more frequently than a placebo or not, whether they work differently from a barbiturate or not — they really do relieve the symptoms of anxiety in a significant proportion of cases.

There is little to guide a physician in selecting one antianxiety drug over another. Few well-controlled comparison trials have been run on these drugs, and "clinical experience does not clearly point to any one of them as outstanding," *The Medical Letter* has noted. "In the absence of a sound basis for a choice, picking a drug for a patient hampered by anxiety must be more or less arbitrary; if one is not effective, or causes unwanted side effects, another can be tried."

There are potential side effects and, indeed, dangers associated with the use of antianxiety drugs. Among the side effects reported for the minor tranquilizers are drowsiness — the most common — and an occasional stomach upset. Allergic reactions, usually consisting of a skin rash, may develop. Bone marrow changes, which normally are reversible when the drug is discontinued, occasionally occur. "In general," the *VA Bulletin* noted, "the disturbances are neither severe nor especially common." Minor side effects appear — and usually soon disappear — early in the course of treatment. Serious disturbances generally disappear when the drug is discontinued.

No doubt drowsiness is a real hazard in patients who drive a car or operate some type of machinery. Lack of coordination can also be a problem. Patients on minor tranquilizers should not drink alcoholic beverages, or take antihistamines or sedatives. Tranquilizers, sedatives, antihistamines, and alcohol all tend to slow reaction time, interfere with muscle coordination, and cause drowsiness. Such effects may be dangerously exaggerated when two or more of those drugs are taken together; and driving becomes even more of a hazard. Some observers see a relationship between widespread use of Librium and Valium and spiraling traffic accident rates. Indeed, the manufacturers of these antianxiety drugs frankly inform physicians that patients receiving Librium and Valium should be cautioned against "hazardous occupations requiring complete mental alertness such as operating machinery or driving a motor vehicle."

Antianxiety drugs are sometimes taken in suicide attempts. Addiction is an occasional hazard. A number of patients take excessive doses of a drug for prolonged periods, and thus become dependent on it. If they discontinue the drug abruptly, serious withdrawal effects may follow.

In December 1967, the Food and Drug Administration (FDA) reported evidence that prolonged high dosage of meprobamate can cause apathy, personality change, depression, stupor, and coma. "Prolonged high dosage" means more than 3,000 miligrams per day for several weeks; a typical tranquilizing dosage is about 1,600 milligrams per day. The FDA has placed meprobamate (Equanil, Miltown) on the list of con-

trolled substances — along with phenobarbital (Luminal), secobarbital (Seconal), and a host of other drugs — under the provisions of the Controlled Substances Act, which replaced the
Drug Abuse Control Amendments to the Food, Drug, and Cosmetic Act. This limits the duration of the prescription and the
number of refills, and requires that records be kept on production and distribution of the drug.

To a great extent, meprobamate has been replaced in general
clinical use by chlordiazepoxide (Librium) and diazepam
(Valium), for which about eighty million prescriptions are
written a year. In August 1973 the more than twenty million
Americans who take these two drugs were put on notice that
chlordiazepoxide and diazepam might join meprobamate on the
controlled substances list; the order took effect in July 1975.

ANTIDEPRESSION DRUGS

While their usefulness is generally conceded, there are differences of opinion on just how useful these drugs are. Dr. Jarvik
commented with respect to the most commonly used of
the antidepression drugs, two of the tricyclics, imipramine
(Tofranil) and amitriptyline (Elavil): "The evidence that
these compounds are of value in the treatment of the various
forms of depression is overwhelming." Dr. Cole, however, was
more cautious. "These drugs generally appear less effective in
carefully controlled clinical studies," he wrote, "than the experience of senior clinical psychiatrists would suggest. In controlled studies, the drugs are usually shown to be better than
placebo, but not dramatically so. Clinicians report generally
more favorable results in ordinary clinical use. From the literature it looks as though six or seven out of ten patients might do
well on imipramine, while four or five out of ten would do
well on inert placebo."

The VA summary was similarly cautious: "Many publications provide eager testimonials for the efficacy of antidepres-

sants, but few of these are based on carefully controlled studies. The Veterans Administration offers the largest number of controlled studies done by any single group. The results support only a lukewarm enthusiasm for these drugs." And again: "It is generally accepted that these drugs are of value. It is doubtful that their value is as great or that their action on depressed patients is as specific as ordinarily thought."

Dr. Jarvik has thus described the major types of depression: "Most individuals have cyclic variations in mood: some sad days are part of the human condition, and it is not the function of the physician to induce perpetual euphoria. Normal individuals will also exhibit marked sadness following the death of a loved one, a major illness, a failure in business, or a severe blow to self-esteem. This response may be so exaggerated or prolonged in a neurotic individual that it becomes incapacitating, but the precipitating factor can usually be identified and the feeling often seems understandable. Such *reactive* (neurotic) depressions may be quite severe and are sometimes prolonged.

"There are still other individuals who seem to have been depressed all of their lives; they seem to find little joy in any form of social interaction, and their self-esteem is chronically low. This picture is common among patients who exhibit alcoholism, narcotic addiction, or sociopathic behavior.

"Another major group consists of those patients whose symptoms have a definite onset, but the onset seems unrelated to significant external events. Such patients are usually older, and the depressions are often considered to be *endogenous* [not brought about by external factors]. Commonly these depressions occur cyclically, and succeeding episodes may be separated by nondepressed periods lasting several months to many years. In this group, the depressive picture is often characterized by marked retardation, feelings of guilt and worthlessness . . . early-morning awakening, decreased appetite, constipation, and weight loss. Still others in this older group may exhibit only a loss of energy and interest associated with a persistent preoccupation with bodily complaints."

Available evidence suggests that antidepression drugs are most effective in relieving the symptoms of endogenous depression. There is also some evidence that they are effective in reactive depressions. There is little if any evidence of their effectiveness in the minor ups and downs of daily life, or in the sadness resulting from an emotional blow, such as the death of a relative.

Unlike antianxiety drugs, antidepression drugs fall into classes with noticeably different effects. Imipramine and amitriptyline are closely related chemically. Although their effects are quite similar, according to the VA summary, "minor differences in efficacy favoring amitriptyline have been found." Side effects (dry mouth and excessive sweating, among other things) are frequent, but these drugs are generally considered relatively safe. Desipramine (Norpramin, Pertofrane) and nortriptyline (Aventyl) are newer drugs, chemically similar to imipramine and amitriptyline. No advantage has been proved for the newer ones, although it is claimed they work faster.

Isocarboxazid (Marplan) and phenelzine (Nardil) are two chemically related drugs known as MAO inhibitors. MAO stands for monoamine oxidase, an enzyme. There is evidence that inhibition of this enzyme is the mechanism by which these drugs exert their effect, although this view has been disputed by some. The MAO inhibitors are less likely to be effective than imipramine or amitriptyline — and are less safe. They are usually prescribed for patients who fail to respond to imipramine or amitriptyline.

Tranylcypromine (Parnate), another MAO inhibitor, was once one of the most popular of the antidepressants. In 1964, however, it was taken off the market for several months because of reports of acute attacks of high blood pressure, sometimes with brain hemorrhage. It was then learned that these side effects were related to the combined effect of tranylcypromine with that of other drugs, or with certain chemicals in foods — especially cheese, such as Roquefort or blue, but also sour cream, chianti, pickled herring, chicken livers, raisins, chocolate, and soy sauce. Tranylcypromine is now back on the market for restricted use. Although it had "some vigorous and vociferous defenders," the VA summary stated, "most of the enthusiasm for this drug is based on anecdotal reports."

Anyone who takes a MAO inhibitor (see table on page 278) must be careful about the simultaneous use of other drugs, including other antidepressants. In addition, you should not begin another kind of antidepressant until at least two weeks after your last dose of a MAO inhibitor, because of the relatively long duration of action of such a drug.

All antidepressants provoke numerous side effects, some mild and frequent, some serious but rare. In certain patients with heart disease, closed-angle type of glaucoma, or an enlarged prostate, these drugs probably should not be used at all.

Frequently, patients will have symptoms of anxiety with depressive features. It may be difficult, if not impossible, for the internist or general practitioner to make a definite diagnosis of either anxiety or depression. Indeed, some patients may require dual treatment. For such people, combinations of antianxiety drugs with antidepressants are available (see table on page 278).

ANTIPSYCHOTIC DRUGS

The first of the major tranquilizers to be introduced, the best known, the most intensively studied, and the most widely used is chlorpromazine, marketed under the brand name Thorazine. It was first used on psychotic patients in 1952. By 1966, according to one estimate, it had been prescribed for at least fifty million patients the world over and ten thousand papers had been published on its actions. Chlorpromazine belongs to a group of chemicals known as the phenothiazines. Many of the other antipsychotic drugs now in common use in the United States — such as trifluoperazine (Stelazine) and fluphenazine (Permitil) — are also phenothiazines, more or less closely resembling chlorpromazine in chemical structure.

Recent additions to the antipsychotic drug group (see table on page 278) include the thioxanthene derivatives (Navane, Taractan); another drug, a butyrophenone (Haldol), is finding increasing favor among clinical psychiatrists. It is also not unusual for certain psychotic patients to be treated with drugs from more than one group — for example, a major tranquilizer and an antidepressant.

A useful adjunct in the treatment of some severely depressed patients is electroconvulsive therapy (ECT) — also called electroshock therapy. Some psychiatrists prefer ECT for patients who may have suicidal tendencies because it offers a more rapid method of relieving depression than drug therapy.

The patients for whom antipsychotic drugs are generally prescribed present a wide variety of symptoms. Among the most common: hallucinations, delusions, belligerence, hostility, paranoia, blunted affect (failure to respond in an appropriate manner to joyous or sad occasions), and emotional withdrawal.

These symptoms may appear in almost any combination; patients who exhibit any of these symptoms to a marked degree may be suffering from schizophrenia, a widespread disorder. Before the advent of the antipsychotic drugs, one-fourth of all hospital beds were occupied by schizophrenics. Tens of thousands of new schizophrenia cases are diagnosed annually.

Skepticism greeted the first reports that chlorpromazine could benefit psychotic patients; there had been too many earlier false alarms. "I urge my colleagues to hurry home and use these new drugs right away — while they still work," one psychiatrist remarked sarcastically at the 1955 convention of the American Psychiatric Association. But the studies of the

VA, NIMH, and other groups no longer leave room for such doubts. Said the VA summary:

"Antipsychotic drugs have a profound beneficial effect on the symptoms of these disorders. This categorical statement is supported by the large-scale controlled trials conducted by the Veterans Administration Cooperative Studies of Chemotherapy in Psychiatry. Using similar techniques, other groups have confirmed these results. The stage of illness matters little; the acutely ill patient in the office and the chronically ill hospitalized patient both improve with drug treatment, differing only in degree. Rarely does a patient treated adequately with an active drug fail to show some degree of improvement, perhaps only minimal symptomatic change, perhaps complete remission of the psychosis."

Early skeptics suspected that the new drugs merely quieted patients and made them more tractable. The VA studies pointed in a different direction: "The inappropriateness of the term 'tranquilizer' is evident when the pattern of response produced by antipsychotic drugs is examined. They certainly do more than simply calm patients or put them in a 'chemical straitjacket.' The core symptoms of schizophrenic reactions are consistently improved...." A collaborative study group of the NIMH reached a similarly impressive conclusion. In their studies, "almost all symptoms and manifestations characteristic of schizophrenic psychoses improved with drug therapy, suggesting that the phenothiazines should be regarded as antischizophrenic in the broad sense."

Neither chlorpromazine nor any of the other antipsychotic drugs "cures" schizophrenia. Patients benefited by these drugs may still show signs of mental or emotional distress. But many who would otherwise require hospitalization are able to live at home. They include patients who had been severely incapacitated by their psychoses, and who are now able, with the help of the drugs, to return to school or college or to earn their living — even at such relatively demanding occupations as teaching and scientific research. "Some patients," Dr. Jarvik added, "are so benefited by the drugs that psychopathology is not detectable even by highly skilled observers."

Antipsychotic drugs have also proved beneficial in the treatment of manic symptoms (a state of excited ebullience accompanied by grandiose ideas, poor judgment, and irritability), chronic brain syndromes, and disorders due to drug or alcohol withdrawals. Chlorpromazine may control agitation and irritability and may help reestablish normal sleep patterns in disturbed elderly patients. Several of the phenothiazines are useful in the control of vomiting, motion sickness, and severe, prolonged hiccups. They also have a variety of important uses in general medicine and surgery.

A new subcategory of antipsychotic drugs, lithium carbonate, has been acclaimed in the lay press as the long-awaited cure for manic-depressive psychosis. Medical authorities agree that lithium has assumed its place among the effective psychotherapeutic drugs, although opinions on its effectiveness vary. Since 1949, when it was first introduced for the treatment of acute mania, many research papers have reported on its use. Only a few of the studies were strictly controlled, but these few did establish that lithium was superior to a placebo in the management of patients with manic-depressive psychosis. Findings vary, however, when lithium is compared to treatment with the major tranquilizers, primarily chlorpromazine. The largest study to date, published in 1971, involved 255 manic patients in eighteen hospitals, and was conducted under the collaborative auspices of the NIMH and the VA. Statistical evaluation of the results of this study suggest the superiority of chlorpromazine over lithium. This conclusion contrasts sharply with the favorable clinical observations in many less well-controlled studies.

Although some authorities contend that chlorpromazine is

superior to lithium in the management of the acutely ill manic patient, it is as a preventive that lithium has probably proven most valuable. Evidence of the safety and effectiveness of the prophylactic use of lithium in preventing recurrences of acute manic states has been demonstrated in a joint VA–NIMH collaborative study.

There is also some evidence, albeit meager, that lithium may have an antidepressant effect and thus can be of some value during depression, as well as during the depressive phase of manic-depressive psychosis. CU's medical consultants believe that definitive evidence on this aspect of lithium action is lacking and that more studies are needed.

Long-term use of lithium has its dangers; patients must remain under close medical supervision. Blood levels of the drug must be monitored, and a close watch maintained for any manifestation of side effects. These may include nodular thyroid enlargement, hypothyroidism, excessive urination due to inability of the kidneys to concentrate urine, elevated white blood cell counts, and an increase in blood sugar. These side effects invariably disappear when use of the drug is stopped.

There is one important advantage of lithium in patient use. The major tranquilizers exert their effect in manic states by depressing the central nervous system, and thus in some patients may promote drowsiness. Lithium, however, produces its benefits without any sedative action. A patient on lithium can usually continue to hold down a job and function capably in society while under treatment.

During the years before 1955, when antipsychotic drugs first came into general use, the number of patients confined in mental hospitals rose each year, reaching a peak of 559,000 by the end of 1955. If the trend had continued, the hospitalized population would have risen to about 793,000 by the end of 1972. Instead, the number each year has fallen more and more rapidly — to 276,000 by the end of 1972. Moreover, the decline in the number of patients *remaining* in mental hospitals was achieved in the face of a notable increase in the number of patients *admitted* to mental hospitals — from 178,000 in 1955 to 461,000 in 1972. The achievement is traceable to a heightened rate of discharge and a shortened average stay (six months in 1955, a little more than one month in 1971).

The VA summary noted, "The vast improvements which have occurred in mental hospitals in the past dozen years would not have been possible without effective drug therapy for the schizophrenic reactions. . . . Once patients consistently improved with drugs, physical facilities could be improved, and hospital personnel could turn their energies from custodial to therapeutic duties. Group therapies, rehabilitation programs, patient self-government, increased patient freedom, and most important, an increased humanity in dealing with patients, all followed."

Equally important, these drugs make it possible for many psychotic patients to receive effective treatment in the psychiatric units of general hospitals near their homes instead of at distant mental hospitals, and for many to be cared for as outpatients by general practitioners or internists as well as by psychiatrists. The result has often been referred to as a "psychiatric revolution."

In an estimated one-third of all cases, a patient who benefits from an antipsychotic drug can in due course — after weeks or months on the drug — discontinue its use without a relapse. But most psychotic patients must continue on the drug for years — and some even for life. NIMH studies have shown that antipsychotic drugs tend to avert relapse when dosage is continued for patients following hospitalization for schizophrenia. For manic-depressive patients, lithium carbonate (as mentioned above) has been demonstrated to prevent relapse, according to results of a joint VA–NIMH multihospital collaborative study begun in 1968. Researchers conducting an ongoing NIMH study at three hospitals in the Baltimore area reported in 1973 on the effectiveness of chlorpromazine (Thorazine): "The effect of drugs in reducing relapse can only be characterized as huge."

A mental health problem of major importance still faces the United States, however. A large proportion of the patients placed on antipsychotic drugs each year fail to continue their medication. The results can be disastrous, as an earlier VA follow-up study had indicated. Following improvement on the drugs, patients were studied over a four-month period in which some continued taking medication, and others discontinued in whole or in part. Results showed that "45 percent of patients who were discontinued showed unmistakable evidence of relapse, as compared with only 5 percent on full doses and fifteen percent on partial doses." Some mental hospitals report that more than half of their admissions are now *readmissions:* Patients do well on the drugs, return home, drop medication, relapse — and must then be readmitted. Conceivably, more community clinics, aftercare clinics, and home visiting services to encourage continuation of medication might prevent many of these rehospitalizations.

The efficacy of long-acting injectable forms of antipsychotic agents, such as fluphenazine, was reported in the *British Medical Journal* in 1973. Patients given these injections need not be burdened with remembering to take their medication each day. Some authorities believe that the procedure may be capable of reducing relapse in schizophrenic patients by 50 percent over the rate achieved with oral dosage. But patient cooperation in returning periodically for injections is an important factor in the success of such programs.

Until recently, because the leading antipsychotic drugs were still protected by patents (see Chapter 30), a patient could not save money by buying them under their generic names. This is no longer true; for example, generic chlorpromazine is now marketed at a considerable saving over its brand-name counter-part, Thorazine. Also, states and cities can buy drugs in large quantities at a fraction of their retail pharmacy prices – an important reason for organizing public drug supply programs.

Antipsychotic drugs are relatively safe. A wide range of side effects, it is true, has been reported for these drugs. Side effects are sufficiently frequent, and some are sufficiently serious, to preclude the use of antipsychotic drugs for calming the minor anxieties of everyday life; but for psychotic patients, the great benefits achieved far outweigh the discomforts of the common side effects and the hazards of the more rare ones.

The most common side effects include such neurological symptoms as slurred speech, a coarse tremor (often in the hands), uncontrollable restlessness, and jerkiness of movement. These drug effects mimic the symptoms of Parkinson's disease, but such symptoms are generally improved by reducing the dosage of the antipsychotic drug, by prescribing a drug used for Parkinson's disease along with the antipsychotic drug, or both. Or the physician may switch the patient over to an anti-psychotic drug of a different type. A relatively permanent, but infrequent, neurological side effect associated with chronic use of phenothiazine antipsychotic drugs is tardive dyskinesia – uncontrollable repetitive movements, usually of the mouth, lips, and tongue.

Many of the other side effects of antipsychotic drugs – such as jaundice which may occur with the phenothiazines – develop early in therapy. Relatively few are likely to be encountered for the first time after months on an effective drug. Hence the fear of future side effects is not a sound reason for discontinu-ing therapy. Reassuring patients on this score, and reminding them that these drugs do *not* lead to addiction, are important public health measures. The fact that these antipsychotic drugs have no addictive properties is significant, because they may be promptly withdrawn should serious side effects develop.

The early recognition of side effects, the VA summary said, remains the best insurance against serious or irreversible effects. Hence, from the practical point of view, in the opinion of CU's medical consultants, patients taking an antipsychotic drug — and their families — should keep four points in mind:

■ The patient should remain under the continuing supervision of a physician, and should return for a checkup periodically— monthly or at least quarterly.

■ If a new side effect is noted, whether or not it seems serious, it should be promptly reported to the physician without waiting for the next scheduled appointment.

■ The patient should scrupulously follow the physician's advice on managing the side effect, *discontinuing the drug only if advised to do so.*

■ Patients on an antipsychotic drug, like those on an antianxiety drug, should drink alcoholic beverages with caution, and should take sedatives or antihistamines only at the direction of a physician familiar with their medical history.

Like antianxiety drugs, antipsychotic drugs can produce drowsiness and other effects likely to impair driving skills and to increase the risk of accidents, either at the wheel or in handling machinery. Yet excessive anxiety and other psychiatric symptoms are also likely to impair skills and increase hazards. As the VA summary pointed out, "one can never be sure whether the person might be more impaired from uncontrollable anxiety than from the drug used to treat it." Actually, antipsychotic drugs, as the VA summary stated, can in many cases "calm the excited or anxious patient without marked impairment of motor function." And "during long-continued treatment, the sedative effects . . . are tolerated remarkably well."

Perhaps the major long-run effect of psychotherapeutic drugs has been a change in public attitude toward mental illness and psychiatric research. When a drug proves capable of abolishing such purely "psychic" symptoms as delusions and hallucinations, the myth of a wall separating the mental from the physical is no longer tenable. Because psychoses can now be viewed as diseases amenable to medication instead of as something "mental," mysterious, and menacing, the attitude toward these illnesses has become healthier.

Major research efforts, moreover, have now been attracted to mental illness. The first fruits of this new research are hardly welcome: a multiplicity of new drugs differing from one another only in minor variations in chemical formula and requiring intensive and costly clinical trials to disprove the excessive initial claims of efficacy and safety made for them. But genuine progress is also being made. The effects on behavior of both chlorpromazine and meprobamate were noted quite by accident; the drugs were developed in the course of searches for drugs having other effects. Now that so many investigators are on the alert for psychotherapeutic drugs, the odds in favor of future significant discoveries are notably improved.

Equally important, improved methods of using the existing antianxiety and antidepression drugs may be developed. The problem at present is that no one can accurately predict which drug is most likely to prove effective in a particular case. If rules for selecting a particular drug to match the needs of a particular patient could be developed, much more would be accomplished with the drugs already available. Studies are under way seeking to classify patients in terms of the drug most likely to prove useful to them.

Finally, these drugs have already cast some light on the possible basis of mental illness — some of the particular cells of the body affected, the enzymes and other chemicals that may be involved, and the nerve pathways implicated. Out of this deeper understanding may yet come drugs having direct and perhaps even curative effects on the underlying diseases.

CU's medical consultants do not believe that psychotherapeutic drugs should be used casually to cope with the vicissitudes of daily living. Some of these drugs take several days, and sometimes weeks, to achieve their effect. The hazards are too great and the likelihood of benefit too small to use psychotherapeutic drugs for a transient case of "the blues." And some authorities believe that these drugs should be used cautiously by those whose anxieties are associated with chronic illness, such as heart disease.

If your physician does prescribe a psychotherapeutic drug, keep in mind the following precautions:

▪ Continuous use of some psychotherapeutic drugs may cause tolerance to develop, and higher dosage may increase the frequency and severity of side effects.

▪ It is important to keep in touch with the physician who has prescribed the drug. Some drugs taken regularly may require periodic blood tests. Even when the medication is used on an intermittent basis (that is, "take when needed"), check back with your physician after several months.

▪ Promptly report all side effects — real or imagined — of any drugs to your physician. Your doctor may wish to reduce the dosage, switch to another drug, or discontinue medication altogether.

▪ When first prescribed a major or minor tranquilizer or an antidepressant, you should not drive or handle machinery until you have ascertained jointly with your physician that drowsiness is not a problem. Drowsiness may be more pronounced with the minor tranquilizers than with any other class of psychotherapeutic drug. You should be aware that reaction time may be impaired and coordination affected by the medication. Such side effects may be reduced by simply lowering the dose or by changing the time of administration. "Since warnings against driving are not often heeded," *The Medical Letter* rea-

Some common psychotherapeutic drugs

Chemical designation	Generic name	Trade name
ANTIANXIETY DRUGS — THE MINOR TRANQUILIZERS		
benzodiazepine derivatives	chlordiazepoxide	Librium*
	diazepam	Valium*
	oxazepam	Serax*
diphenylmethane derivatives	hydroxyzine	Atarax, Vistaril
glycerol derivatives	meprobamate	Equanil,* Miltown*
	tybamate	Solacen, Tybatran
ANTIDEPRESSION DRUGS		
MAO inhibitors	isocarboxazid	Marplan
	phenelzine	Nardil
	tranylcypromine	Parnate
tricyclic derivatives	amitriptyline	Elavil
	desipramine	Norpramin, Pertofrane
	imipramine	Tofranil
	nortriptyline	Aventyl
ANTIPSYCHOTIC DRUGS		
The Major Tranquilizers		
butyrophenones	haloperidol	Haldol
phenothiazine derivatives	chlorpromazine	Thorazine
	fluphenazine	Permitil
	perphenazine	Trilafon
	trifluoperazine	Stelazine
thioxanthene derivatives	chlorprothixene	Taractan
	thiothixene	Navane
Antimanic Drugs		
lithium	lithium carbonate	Eskalith, Lithane, Lithonate
COMBINATION DRUGS		
tricyclic derivative and phenothiazine derivative	amitriptyline and perphenazine	Etrafon, Triavil

*Subject to the Controlled Substances Act of 1970.

sons, "the physician should avoid unnecessary prescription of drugs."

Other drugs are also likely to increase driving hazards. Sedatives, narcotics, and many antihistamines, including the ones used in cold remedies and in motion sickness remedies, may similarly induce drowsiness or impair alertness and muscle coordination.

■ If you take any psychotherapeutic drug, you should severely limit your intake of alcoholic beverages, barbiturates, or any other drug that induces drowsiness, such as antihistamines, unless your physician says it is all right. Ingesting two of these kinds of substances (for example, a tranquilizer and alcohol) may, in many people, produce a synergistic effect. In other words, one's response to the combination of drugs may be greater than that produced by either drug alone — what can be termed "a 1 + 1 = 3 effect."

Chapter 26

How to evaluate news about "miracles"

IN ADDITION to the constant barrage of drug advertising which many people have learned to disregard, there are subtler attacks from drug publicity posing as news. Hardly a magazine appears on the stands without one or more medical articles; newspapers run medical columns and medical news; there is a steady outpouring of medical books for lay readers; and television and radio convey medical information not only in news and documentary programs but in programs like "Medical Center" and "Marcus Welby, M.D."

Some of this material is more or less accurate and helpful; a great deal of it is not. Much of what we read, see, and hear about medicine is inspired (and sometimes subsidized) by the publicity staffs of drug companies.

Drug publicity may go out under the firm's name, or it may issue from a "medical information bureau," a "medical news service," or some similar cover name designed to impress readers, writers, television producers, and editors — and, possibly, to obscure the backing of drug manufacturers. The objective is to get news of the product into newspapers and magazines and on radio and television. The theory — and it apparently works — is that if people hear about new drugs they will rush to their doctors' offices and demand them. Newspapers often publish promotion releases without distinguishing between what is scientifically valuable and what is pure promotional puffery. In magazines, a story may be signed by a free-lance or staff writer, but it is often inspired by a drug manufacturer's publicity bureau which has steered the writer to a researcher doing work for the company on one of its products. Some companies even subsidize the writing of free-lance articles later sold to magazines. The claims made in these articles often bear little or no relation to actual performance; indeed, some overly optimistic articles are based largely on what investigators *hope* they will find in research just getting under way.

The family doctor, who should be in a position to help patients appraise the optimistic press reports, rarely has time to keep abreast of the steady flow of literature appearing in legitimate medical journals — let alone quasi-medical articles in the popular press. Even for a physician who keeps up with medical news, there are "detail men" to contend with — salesmen hired by drug companies to promote the products they sell. Most of the large companies employ many hundreds of these salesmen, and they subject doctors to heavy sales pressure. The Council on Economic Priorities reports that in 1972 drug companies spent about $1 billion on promotion — the equivalent of $5,000 per doctor. And detail men represent about 70 percent of the promotional budget.

Under regulations of the Food and Drug Administration (FDA) manufacturers may not issue promotional material representing that a drug is safe or effective before the drug has been approved by the FDA. However, news reports may be circulated during the trial period, and it is entirely possible that such reports are partisan and misleading, even if they are not untrue.

Much pharmaceutical research is simply the offspring of competitive pressure. Many "new" products come out each year without regard to specific need for them in medical practice; only a few can be considered real advances in therapy. Most new products are in direct competition with older drugs made by other pharmaceutical companies. Sometimes a new drug is actually the same old drug, only with new use indications. Or established medications are sometimes combined, and the combination advertised to physicians as "new." Variations in the chemical formula of an old medication occasionally bring real improvement in a drug's action, or tone down some serious side effect. More often, a new formulation has little additional value except to the company holding the patent.

Many of the new forms and chemical variations go through a series of "research" stages; at each stage encouraging results are likely to be reported in the general press as well as in professional journals. In fact, most of these news stories herald a business coup, on a par with a paint company's discovery of a way to obtain a new shade of blue. Occasionally, a story may be planted at a strategic time to manipulate the stock of a drug manufacturer.

The prudent, therefore, can protect themselves to some extent by approaching medical news with full awareness that the profit motive stimulates the promotion and marketing of many new drugs. How can you judge a particular piece of news? It usually helps to ask yourself the following six questions. None of the answers may be decisive, but taken all together they can be indicative of the value of the drug.

1. WHAT IS THE SOURCE OF THE STORY? An announcement from one of the National Institutes of Health or from a major medical center is more likely to be significant than one from the laboratories of a drug firm, however prominent.

2. WHO PAID FOR THE STUDY? Be very critical of the source of funding for the research. Even though some pharmaceutical companies do indeed contribute funds for worthwhile basic research, experimental studies sponsored by drug firms must

always be interpreted cautiously or suspected of bias. The same goes for research sponsored by other commercial interests whose motivation for funding studies may be equally self-serving. If government-funded, the research might be valid — or it might not. On some levels of government, political purposes may be served by the premature release of research findings. And the validity of research may be imperiled by changes in policy, which can lead to the elimination or reduction of funds for promising projects. Nevertheless, with government funding, there is more likelihood of disinterest and impartiality. Competition for research grants can be intense, and awards are usually made to dependable investigators with promising projects.

Somewhat more reliable as sources of disinterested research are major private foundations (such as Rockefeller or Whitney) that award grants and scholarships to scientists. National health organizations (such as American Heart Association or American Cancer Society) also sponsor worthwhile research related to their areas of interest. These groups provide many highly qualified investigators with support for quality research in fields allied to the basic interests of the sponsoring organization.

3. WHAT STAGE OF RESEARCH IS BEING REPORTED — TEST TUBE, ANIMAL, OR HUMAN? Drug research usually takes place on several different levels of experimentation. A drug's chemical reactions and structural modifications at the molecular level are the particular concerns of basic science. In the next stage, the pharmacological action of the drug on organisms is studied either at the cellular level (which includes viruses and bacteria) or in multicellular organisms (such as rodents and mammals). Animal experimentation can be scaled to varying degrees of complexity, ranging from the use of lower animals, such as rats, to more sophisticated studies with primates. Naturally, the more highly developed the experimental model, the more clini-

cally applicable to humans should be the results of a study. With drugs that have selective pharmacological action, the organ affected, whether the liver, heart, or kidney, can be removed from the animal and studied as isolated tissue. Only after a drug has been thoroughly studied — not only for physiological effects but also for toxicity — should human experimentation be considered. The final step, clinical testing, involves administering the test drug to human beings, according to the provisions of a well-designed protocol approved by the FDA.

Each stage of drug research has its own significance, but the results do not necessarily carry over from one stage to the next. For example, the effects of the drug being studied on isolated rat liver in the test tube may be observed and measured. When the same drug is given to a live rat, however, the effects may not be similar to those noted in vitro. The rat liver in its normal anatomic setting is affected by multiple factors which may reinforce, distort, or otherwise alter the action of the drug under study. Clinical testing is more complicated still. Human beings are more complex than laboratory animals, as well as chemically different in some respects. Furthermore, people have highly developed nervous systems, hence emotions and feelings, which affect them in elaborate and as yet poorly understood ways.

4. HOW VALID WERE THE CLINICAL TESTING PROCEDURES? A large proportion of what passes for clinical research is merely old-fashioned trial and error, the results of which are highly vulnerable to false deductions. The reasoning is simple: A drug is given to a sick person; the patient becomes well; therefore the drug is responsible for the cure. The observation that the sick person became well may be accurate, but the deduction that the drug was responsible for the improvement may be false. Illness very often is self-limited — healing or improvement often occurs spontaneously, whether or not medication is used.

Even with sound testing procedures, researchers face additional hazards in clinical trials of drugs. The so-called placebo effect is a well-known phenomenon. As many as 40 percent of participants in some studies report relief of their symptoms when dummy medication has been administered.

Furthermore, results can be distorted by both patient enthusiasm and investigator bias. Just about every sick person wants to get well, and even the most detached investigator wants to come up with a successful result. Both are influenced, perhaps unconsciously, to give the benefit of a doubt to the success of the treatment under study.

Careful investigators attempt to neutralize such factors by resorting to a controlled study — the sound and long-established way to prove or disprove the value of a new medication or treatment. One group of patients receives the drug being tested, and a similar group receives a placebo which looks exactly like the test drug. This method may also utilize a double-blind procedure, in which the drug and the placebo are independently coded so that neither the patients nor the people who administer them and record the results know who receives the drug and who does not. The code is not broken until the study is finished. In addition, the random selection of patients for such tests is important. The experimental and control groups should then be well matched in terms of age, sex, and other important variables. Crossover studies, in which drug and placebo are switched without knowledge of patient or observer, also add considerably to test validity.

5. HOW EXTENSIVE WAS THE TEST? Of significance here are the number of test subjects, the length of follow-up study of the patients to see how permanent any positive results might be, and the duration of continued dosage if the drug is for long-term use. The greater each of these has been, the more likely it is that the results will stand up with the passage of time. In this respect it is important to remember that a single study is just that. Ask yourself whether the results of the study have been

corroborated by other disinterested investigators.

6. WHAT DOES THE STORY REPORT ABOUT RESULTS AND ABOUT SIDE EFFECTS? How complete was the cure or relief? Were there risks or side effects and, if so, how serious were they? How do the benefits of the new drug or treatment compare with those of standard measures already in use? Were the benefits temporary or long-lasting?

Clear answers to the questions discussed above will help you to evaluate news about drugs, devices, or medical procedures, and to decide whether the label of "miracle" is really warranted.

Chapter 27

Cortisone: the "wonder" hormone

IN RECENT YEARS hopes have been raised among the sick (and their families) by popular accounts of the "miracles" performed by cortisone, an adrenal steroid hormone, and its modern analogues, chiefly prednisone. These drugs, in doses considerably greater than normal human adrenal gland production, are remarkably effective in relieving symptoms of rheumatic, allergic, and related disorders; certain skin and blood abnormalities; and even some varieties of cancer.

The dramatic nature of the relief – plus the fact that the extraction, identification, and synthesis of adrenal steroid hormones have constituted one of the triumphs of pharmaceutical research – has led to widespread, perhaps inordinate publicity. Magazines and newspapers have so often hailed cortisone as a "wonder" drug that many patients have an exaggerated view of what it can do.

Adrenal steroid hormones are one type of the body's many internal secretions produced by specialized endocrine or ductless glands. These glands secrete their hormones and other active chemicals directly into the bloodstream in response to stimuli from various parts of the body. In general, hormones either facilitate or inhibit certain types of chemical action in the body. It has been customary to think of each hormone as exerting one specific action — insulin affecting sugar metabolism, for example. However, while it is true that each hormone acts predominantly on a specific tissue, recent research indicates that the influence of each one is wider than was formerly believed. This change obviously makes a big difference when hormones are used in amounts in excess of the normal rate of production in human beings, and especially if such dosage is prolonged, as is often the case in a chronically ill patient. The effects on tissues other than the specific target of the hormone may prove to be dangerous — or they may be just what is needed.

Adrenal steroid hormones are produced by the outer layer or *cortex* (hence the names *cort*isone and *cort*icosteroid) of the adrenal glands, which are situated atop each kidney. Knowledge of these glands dates back many years, and researchers have identified more than forty different hormones or active chemicals produced by adrenal cortex tissue. Adrenal steroid hormones may be divided into three groups, according to their main action.

Perhaps the most important class of adrenal steroid hormones is the glucocorticoids (hydrocortisone is the major one produced by the human adrenals), which control various aspects of body metabolism affecting protein, fats, and carbohydrates. A second class of hormones, called mineralocorticoids (of which aldosterone is the most active metabolically), controls the sodium content of urine, sweat, and saliva by acting mainly on the kidneys and also on the sweat and salivary glands. And third, other hormones called sex steroids are produced by the adrenal cortex, although in far less amounts, under normal circumstances, than the sex steroids produced by the testes and the ovaries.

Even before the various adrenal hormones were isolated and identified, extracts of whole adrenal tissue were used to treat primary adrenal insufficiency, known as Addison's disease. (For a discussion of adrenal insufficiency, see Chapter 20.) Formerly, this disease was frequently caused by destruction of the adrenal glands by tuberculosis. Now, however, cases of this *rare* disorder are most often due to the gradual atrophy of both adrenal glands without evidence of infection. Current theory holds that, for reasons as yet unknown, victims of Addison's disease develop antibodies to their own adrenal tissue — antibodies which eventually destroy both adrenal glands. Investigation has shown that the blood serum of patients with Addison's disease contains antibodies that react against human adrenal tissue. The name that is given to this disease process is autoimmunity. Such common ailments as pernicious anemia and certain types of hypothyroidism are also autoimmune diseases. Addison's disease is treatable by simple replacement doses (equivalent to what normal adrenals produce) of synthetic adrenal steroid hormones.

Broader experimentation with adrenal steroid hormones started when the hormones became available in fairly large quantities. Cortisone (Cortone) — a derivative of the major glucocorticoid, hydrocortisone (Cortef, Hydrocortone) — was partially synthesized in 1946; within two years a commercially feasible process for its manufacture had been worked out. In 1948, Dr. Philip S. Hench and his colleagues at the Mayo Clinic reported a radically new concept, the first nonendocrine use of a hormone. The doctors had given the drug to patients who were badly crippled with rheumatoid arthritis. Almost without exception, these patients were relieved, at least for a time, of pain and tenderness in the affected joints, and many of them regained a degree of motion they had not known for years. It was soon apparent that in this disease cortisone was not correcting a deficiency, but that it acted in some way on the inflammatory process. Although less dramatic results in more extensive and longer tests and the appearance of a variety of undesirable side effects have dimmed the optimism aroused by its first successes, Dr. Hench's report marked the beginning of cortisone's career as a "wonder" drug.

Despite the fact that the precise mechanism of action of adrenal steroid hormones on tissue inflammation has not yet been fully worked out, their ability to reduce inflammation, as well as their ability to affect the immune mechanism, has led to their use in a variety of disorders. In addition to helping many patients with rheumatoid arthritis, steroid hormone treatment has proved to be helpful in relieving the symptoms of rheumatic fever, lupus erythematosus, sarcoidosis, nephrosis, ulcerative colitis, asthma, and other diseases.

Incorporated into creams and ointments, cortisone and its more recently synthesized analogues, such as triamcinolone (Aristocort, Kenacort), are effective in relieving inflammation and itching in certain types of acute and chronic eczema and in some allergic skin disorders. In itching of the anal region or vulva for which no specific cause can be found or which is seemingly psychogenic, the use of a corticosteroid hormone ointment may be more effective than any other topical agent. And in one serious skin disease, pemphigus, corticosteroids taken by mouth not only relieve symptoms but may prolong life for many years.

Topical corticosteroids in the form of eye drops have also proved of great value in treating certain acute inflammations of the eye, such as allergic conjunctivitis and iritis. Here the steroids help to keep inflammatory reactions within bounds. However, special care must be exercised in their use because of their tendency to increase pressure in the eye (see Chapter 6). And at least one severe disorder of the eye, herpes simplex infection, can be seriously aggravated by use of these hormones.

In treating some severe blood and bone marrow disorders, steroids have proved effective in temporarily halting or controlling these diseases. In such instances, the hormones prolong life or make life more comfortable, rather than save it. In some types of acute hemolytic anemia, corticosteroid hormones can sometimes be lifesaving — by controlling the destruction of red blood cells.

Less spectacular, but still important to the sufferer, is the use of corticosteroid hormones in the treatment of bursitis and tendonitis. Suspensions of the hormones, injected directly into the inflamed joints, may be of value in reducing pain and tenderness, and they may restore movement sooner than older methods of treatment.

Despite some failures, the long list of more-or-less dramatic successes in the use of corticosteroids has led to considerable overenthusiasm. A major problem resulting from the reception accorded these drugs has been the failure to recognize sufficiently the other side of the story. For instance, some uses of the hormones are of dubious value. These include their incorporation into various shotgun preparations (see page 32) containing antibiotics, antihistamines, and topical anesthetics, and their use with other drugs in nose and eye drops, suppositories, and sprays variously intended for colds, sinusitis, or hemorrhoids. Undesirable and sometimes serious side effects have always been a problem in therapy with adrenal steroid hormones.

Serious complications include stomach and duodenal ulceration with bleeding, changes in behavior, decreased resistance to infection, thinning of the bones (osteoporosis), and triggering of latent diabetes. Another unwanted effect from long-term use (over a period of months) is a quite natural physiological phenomenon. When cortisone (or one of its analogues) is taken regularly, the pituitary's ability to produce ACTH (adrenocorticotropic hormone) is reduced, and the natural stimulus to normal functioning of the adrenal cortex is removed. Thus, with long-term corticosteroid treatment, the adrenal cortex gradually shrinks from lack of stimulation, and the body's ability to produce its own adrenal cortical hormones is drastically reduced. Should the prescribed steroid medication be stopped inadvertently because of a patient's inability to communicate the need for medication following a serious accident or stroke, the result could be life-threatening. Therefore every patient on long-term therapy with this type of drug should carry the information where it is readily available — on a wallet card or bracelet, for example. In the event of an emergency operation or a serious accident, supplementary doses of the hormone may be required.

The most common and one of the most serious problems in treatment with adrenal steroid hormones is retention of sodium by the kidneys, leading to elevation of blood pressure and edema (swelling of the tissues with water).* Prednisone (Meticorten, Servisone), the first analogue of cortisone to be developed, does not have this drawback. In the opinion of CU's medical consultants, other synthetic analogues of cortisone, such as betamethasone (Celestone), dexamethasone (Decadron, Hexadrol), or prednisolone (Meticortelone, Sterane), offer little in the way of advantages over prednisone, and are more expensive.

It should be remembered that the inflammatory and allergic responses subdued by adrenal steroid hormones are normal and necessary defenses of the body. It is legitimate to question whether these defenses should be interfered with by broad systemic treatment except when a severe inflammatory or allergic disorder proves markedly limiting to one's well-being, activity, and long-range health. This question is particularly pertinent when there are other treatments for the disorder which, in some cases at least, may be as good as hormone therapy. In rheumatoid arthritis, for example, controlled studies

* The use of a diuretic to offset water retention must be carefully supervised. Since both diuretics and corticosteroids may cause a loss of potassium from the body, when both drugs are used together the effect may be compounded. Liquid potassium replacements are usually prescribed to prevent potassium depletion.

have indicated that, from the standpoint of long-range treatment, plain old-fashioned aspirin therapy is preferable. Aspirin is almost as effective as corticosteroids in relieving symptoms and permitting activity (see Chapter 19). It is also far safer to use and a good deal less expensive.

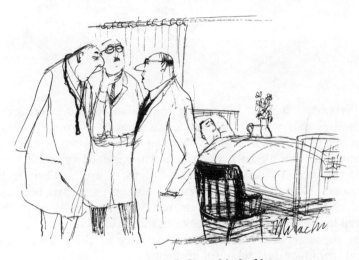

"Then we're agreed. *Some* kind of bug
has bit him."

Chapter 28

The other side of antibiotics

ANTIBIOTICS have eliminated or controlled so many infectious diseases that virtually everyone has benefited from their use at one time or another. Even without such personal experience, however, one would have to be isolated indeed to be unaware of the virtues — real and alleged — of these drugs. Their truly remarkable success in the chemical war on germs has been extensively reported by the press, television, and radio. And any gap in the media accounts has been more than compensated for by the aggressive public relations activity of the pharmaceutical manufacturers who sell antibiotics.

In contrast, the inadequacies and potential dangers of these remarkable drugs are much less widely known. And the lack of such knowledge can be unfortunate, especially if it leads patients to pressure their doctors into prescribing antibiotics when such medication is not really needed, or if it leads them to switch from one doctor to another until they find one who is, so to speak, antibiotics-minded. An October 1973 article in the *Journal of the American Medical Association (JAMA)* reported that a study had shown that in a single year about one of every four persons in the United States received penicillin and that 90 percent of the drug usage was unnecessary.

Because the positive side of the antibiotics story is so well known, it seems more useful here to review some of the immediate and long-range problems that can result from indiscriminate use of these drugs. It should be understood that calamities from the use of antibiotics are rare in proportion to the enormous amounts of these potent drugs being administered to patients. But the potential hazards, so little touched on generally, do need greater emphasis.

Almost all antibiotics are prescription drugs. A few antibiotics, however, are permitted in such over-the-counter (OTC) products as nasal sprays, lozenges, troches, creams, and ointments. Even if these products do no harm — a claim that can be questioned, especially in regard to the development of resistant germs (discussed below) — there is no benefit whatsoever in using them. If you have an infection serious enough to warrant the launching of chemical warfare, you need antibiotics in a form and dosage prescribed by a physician, and not in nonprescription products for self-medication. Even small amounts of an OTC antibiotic ointment can cause an allergic skin reaction.

Antibiotics are far from being a sure cure-all. There are wide gaps in their ability to master contagious diseases. Such important viral infections as the common cold and infectious hepatitis still await conquest. In fact, little progress has been made in the chemotherapy of most viruses.

Bacteria, along with viruses, are responsible for most common infections. Two general types of bacteria are distinguished according to the color they show when smeared on a glass slide, treated with a chemical known as Gram's stain, and then viewed under a microscope. Bacteria that retain the stain are termed "Gram-positive," while those that do not are called "Gram-negative."

Antibiotics that act exclusively on just Gram-positive or on just Gram-negative bacteria are known as narrow-spectrum antibiotics. Examples of narrow-spectrum antibiotics include penicillin, erythromycin, and lincomycin (which attack mostly Gram-positive organisms), and colistin and gentamicin (which attack Gram-negative organisms). Broad-spectrum antibiotics such as ampicillin and tetracycline are capable of handling infections caused by either Gram-positive *or* Gram-negative bacteria — or even mixed infections, such as those occurring in certain wounds, involving both types of bacteria. In certain cases of mixed infections, the use of two narrow-spectrum antibiotics (one Gram-positive and one Gram-negative) may be preferable to the use of a single broad-spectrum antibiotic.

Antibiotics in general can also be classified as bacteriostatic or bactericidal. Bacteriostatic antibiotics, such as tetracycline, prevent multiplication of the bacterial population and allow natural body mechanisms to take over and heal the infection. Bactericidal antibiotics, such as penicillin, actually destroy the organism. When an exact diagnosis has been made, and the choice of antibiotics is between one that is bacteriostatic or one that is bactericidal, the latter is preferred.

In time, certain bacteria become resistant to antibiotics. Because of the widespread use of antibiotics that destroy Gram-positive bacteria, Gram-negative types are assuming increasing clinical importance. At least one researcher has estimated that Gram-negative bacteria cause serious infections in about 1 percent of patients in hospitals and result in the death of about 100,000 Americans each year.

It has been well established that the increase in strains of bacteria resistant to a particular antibiotic correlates directly with inadequate dosage and inappropriate use. For example, one hospital survey showed that before erythromycin was widely used there, all strains of staphylococci found in patients and staff personnel were sensitive to this antibiotic's action. When doctors at the hospital started extensive use of erythromycin, however, resistant staphylococcal strains began to appear.

The development of bacterial resistance can be minimized by

more discriminating use of antibiotics. When an antibiotic must be used, the best way to prevent the development of resistance is to wipe out the infection rapidly and thoroughly. It is of utmost importance that adequate dosage be taken by the patient. The doctor chooses the drug, but the patient must be responsible for completing the full course of the recommended treatment, even though the symptoms should disappear before the prescribed medication has all been taken.

Physicians and the general public had accepted antibiotics so enthusiastically that some drug manufacturers devised a scheme for broadening sales by using more than one antibiotic in their formulations. The practice became so widespread that these medications earned a special designation, "piggyback" antibiotics. The name refers to the addition of a second antibiotic — one just along for the ride — on top of an antibiotic appropriate for an illness. Most authorities agree that piggyback antibiotics — fixed-combination medications — are irrational. Few infections call for more than one antibiotic. Even on the rare occasions when a second antibiotic might be indicated, these formulations frequently include it in inadequate dosage. The amount of each antibiotic and duration of treatment should be specifically tailored by the doctor to the patient.

Consider Panalba, a fixed-combination medication with two antibiotics, tetracycline and novobiocin. Each capsule contained 250 milligrams of the former and 125 milligrams of the latter. Usual dosage was four capsules a day, totaling 1,000 milligrams of tetracycline and 500 of novobiocin. While 1,000 milligrams of tetracycline would be considered by many physicians to be an adequate daily dosage of this antibiotic, 500 milligrams of novobiocin would not be. (In fact, today novobiocin is not widely recommended. *AMA Drug Evaluations* states: "Novobiocin is not the drug of first or second choice for any infection.")

Panalba, manufactured by Upjohn, first appeared in the late

1950s; large-scale promotion made it an immediate sales hit. It became one of the 200 most prescribed drugs, racking up during its heyday an estimated $16 to $20 million a year in sales. After a National Academy of Sciences–National Research Council (NAS–NRC) panel found that Panalba did not do what the manufacturer claimed it would, the Food and Drug Administration (FDA) forced its removal from the market in 1970. Possibly the most damaging evidence against it came from studies in the manufacturer's own files. An FDA medical officer concluded, after reviewing the files, that each of Panalba's components would have entered the bloodstream at a higher level if each had been given individually. "This," he added, "would serve to defeat any purposeful effectiveness the two drugs may have had in combination and certainly leaves a great doubt whether this combination has ever been more or even as effective as tetracycline alone . . ."

After the Panalba decision, the FDA publicized a list of 350 prescription and OTC drugs judged "ineffective," and a second list of more than 150 characterized as only "possibly effective." Many of the drugs were combinations of antibiotics; it is this kind of "shotgun" remedy (see page 32) that CU's medical consultants advise against.

In general, antibiotics — especially penicillin, cephalosporin, and neomycin — are among the more frequent sensitizing agents in human beings. Allergic reactions to antibiotics can vary from mild to life-threatening. The most severe reaction — sometimes fatal — is known as anaphylactic shock. It most commonly follows injection of an antibiotic — especially penicillin. According to the October 1973 *JAMA* article, it has been estimated that not more than twenty-five of every ten million penicillin injections lead to "serious consequences." But of those twenty-five injections, three may result in death.

Anaphylactic shock can also be caused by bee stings (see page 133). Indeed, on rare occasions, it may follow injection of virtually any substance. Within minutes of taking the offending medication — usually a penicillin injection — the patient begins to experience difficulty in breathing, accompanied by a tight feeling in the chest and possibly by severe generalized itching. Collapse and death may follow; life-saving treatment consists of an immediate injection of adrenaline followed by an antihistamine. This severe reaction happens much less frequently when an antibiotic is taken by mouth. CU's medical consultants urge all patients to wait ten minutes in the doctor's office or clinic after receiving an injection of penicillin to make sure that if anaphylactic shock does occur, immediate treatment is available.

Anaphylactic shock usually happens without warning, often in a patient who has no history of penicillin allergy. Fortunately, anaphylactic shock is uncommon. The more typical allergic reaction to penicillin takes the form of a generalized itchy rash or hives, which usually develops during the time the medication is being taken or up to two weeks following discontinuance. The rash may persist from several days to a week or more and may cause severe discomfort. The allergic reaction itself is best treated by an antihistamine; in severe cases, corticosteroids may be necessary. Itching may be helped by the use of analgesics, such as aspirin or acetaminophen, as well as by cool cornstarch baths.

It is unlikely that someone using a drug for the very first time will develop an allergic reaction to it. However, the initial contact with the sensitizing drug may have been inadvertent. For example, many years ago penicillin was used by the brewing industry to prevent bacterial contamination in the fermenting process. And some beer drinkers may have received a small sensitizing dose of penicillin along with their brew. Thus some subsequent exposure to penicillin — say, as medication — could precipitate an allergic reaction in sensitized beer drinkers.

The interval between the time of initial exposure and the first allergic reaction may be as short as a few days or may extend over several years. For reasons that are as yet unclear, an individual can become sensitized and have an allergic reaction after many uneventful exposures to an antibiotic. Once an allergy to a medication has been well documented, it would seem prudent to avoid that medication. Also possible is an allergic reaction to an antibiotic similar in chemical structure to one that is a known allergen for that patient. Thus a patient who is sensitive to penicillin may show an allergic reaction to cephalosporin. In fact, an additional objection to piggyback antibiotics is the unnecessary exposure of the patient to double the allergic potential of just a single antibiotic.

Skin tests that would help determine which individuals are prone to allergic reactions have still not been perfected. To minimize the risk of anaphylactic shock in illnesses in which penicillin is the preferred treatment, a doctor questions the patient carefully about previous allergic reactions to drugs. In case of doubt, another antibiotic may be substituted.

Other untoward reactions to antibiotics may be troublesome. A sore mouth, a "furry" tongue, cramps, diarrhea, anal itch, nausea, vomiting, and so on, occur most frequently after oral use of a broad-spectrum antibiotic, most commonly tetracycline. (For the reason why tetracycline should not be taken toward the end of pregnancy, see page 234.) These reactions may result from direct irritative effects of the antibiotic on the stomach and the intestines, or from elimination by the antibiotic of harmless bacteria normally found in the gastrointestinal tract. With the natural balance of power destroyed, antibiotic-resistant staphylococci and fungi, which are also normally present, are free to flourish and cause what is called a superinfection. Such infections can be quite debilitating and difficult to cure.

In women taking broad-spectrum antibiotics, growth of the

yeast monilia can cause a most distressing vaginal itch for which treatment may be difficult. In an attempt to prevent this unpleasant complication, one pharmaceutical company, Squibb, came up with a new kind of piggyback antibiotic, Mysteclin-F. In a single capsule this drug combined tetracycline in usual doses with amphotericin B, an antibiotic added ostensibly to prevent infection by monilia. In 1969 the NAS–NRC, in a statement to the FDA, declared that Mysteclin-F was ineffective as a fixed combination. According to the panel report, it would be preferable to prescribe adequate amounts of an antifungal drug when clinically indicated rather than to use a drug indiscriminately. However, Mysteclin-F is still sold by Squibb, but with the addition of a warning label, required by the FDA, which quotes the panel's finding that the drug is ineffective. As of this writing, Mysteclin-F is still being prescribed.

If a vaginal infection by monilia should develop during treatment with an antibiotic, it is much better, in the opinion of CU's medical consultants, to treat the vaginal itch with adequate amounts of an antifungal agent such as nystatin (Mycostatin) in the form of intravaginal inserts.

A few antibiotics have such toxic effects that their usefulness is strictly limited. They include such relatively new Gram-negative drugs as gentamicin and kanamycin, which can sometimes cause deafness as well as impairment of kidney function.

The story of chloramphenicol is well known to readers of CONSUMER REPORTS. As Chloromycetin (its Parke, Davis trade name), this drug enjoyed great popularity in the 1950s. Its indiscriminate use for minor infections resulted in several well-publicized fatalities due to aplastic anemia, a disease of the bone marrow in which blood-forming elements are suppressed. Aplastic anemia is relatively rare. But with the use of Chloromycetin, according to a California study, the risk of death from aplastic anemia increases dramatically.

One kind of aplastic anemia resulting from the use of chloramphenicol is irreversible and inevitably fatal. This hypersensitivity reaction of the bone marrow to chloramphenicol is not related to the amount of the drug taken and may follow the administration of even very small quantities. Fortunately, this phenomenon is rare. The more common type of aplastic anemia following use of chloramphenicol *is* dose-related, and therefore is usually reversible once the drug has been discontinued. However, it is impossible to predict which type of aplastic anemia could occur in an individual who takes chloramphenicol.

While fatal bone marrow failure as a direct result of using chloramphenicol is unlikely (occurring about once in approximately 40,000 to 80,000 patients), the odds hardly ever need be risked. Chloromycetin is rarely the drug of choice for any disease, especially with the emergence of newer antibiotics. Medical authorities who testified at Senate hearings in 1969 estimated that about 90 to 99 percent of Chloromycetin therapy was uncalled for. Yet the same product is still widely promoted and prescribed today, with just one change. The label now includes warnings that "serious and fatal" blood conditions are known to occur after administration of the drug. Label warnings are reasonably complete for the Parke, Davis product distributed in the United States. However, a recent study prepared for the International Organization of Consumers Unions found that label warnings are seriously deficient for chloramphenicol marketed abroad, where antibiotics and other drugs can frequently be obtained without a doctor's prescription. That organization has called for standardization of label warnings and stricter control of international distribution.

Obviously, an antibiotic with potentially dangerous side effects should be used only when it is specifically indicated and when no safer antibiotic is available for the same purpose. A physician's selection of an antibiotic may be influenced by testing the infecting organism for its susceptibility to various antibiotics. It is usually possible to detect the infecting organism by means of a bacteriological smear and culture. In the case of a respiratory infection or pneumonia, this may be done by a throat or sputum culture. Similarly, infected wounds, urine, and stools may be cultured. When, in the course of a day or two, growth of the organism is noted on the culture medium, its susceptibility to various antibiotics may be tested and reported in order of effectiveness. The doctor then chooses the most effective antibiotic with the least side effects.

Another factor that might influence the physician's choice of an antibiotic is the site of the infection. For example, for an infection in the urinary tract the physician may prescribe an antibiotic that is excreted in high amounts in the urine. In some instances, the cost of a particular antibiotic might be the determining factor when a choice exists among several drugs with near-equal efficacy. The cost to the patient of various antibiotics may often be less if the physician prescribes a drug by its generic name rather than by its brand name (see Chapter 30).

The expense and the possible troubles that can result from antibiotic treatment should not keep anyone from using one of these drugs when it is clearly necessary. Nor should the possibility of such problems discourage certain preventive uses of antibiotics, which have proved extremely valuable.

Actually, there are relatively few occasions that call for the use of an antibiotic as a prophylactic medication — that is, to prevent an illness from occurring. More often than not, these drugs are misused when taken prophylactically. The most common misuse is their administration in the course of a common cold, ostensibly to prevent secondary infection. Not only does such use of an antibiotic often result in the emergence of resistant strains of bacteria, but it was probably totally unnecessary in the first place. The vast majority of colds are self-limited and do not progress to bacterial complications.

In patients with known rheumatic heart disease, however, antibiotics *should* be used prophylactically prior to, during, and after dental extractions or drilling of cavities, the birth of a baby, and operations on the gastrointestinal or genitourinary tract. Such antibiotic prophylaxis can prevent subacute bacterial endocarditis, a disease that is always serious and sometimes fatal.

In addition, young patients who have had one or more attacks of rheumatic fever, may be able to avoid recurrences — which could result in new or further heart damage — with daily administration of prophylactic doses of penicillin, continued well into adult life. (Erythromycin is a reasonable alternative in cases of penicillin allergy.) The incidence of rheumatic fever has been declining, no doubt as a result of prompt recognition and treatment of streptococcal sore throats, which bear a causal relationship to acute rheumatic fever. Treatment of such sore throats usually consists of a ten-day course of penicillin.

People whose sexual partners are being treated for either gonorrhea or syphilis should consult a physician or a clinic for prophylactic treatment with an appropriate antibiotic. Another indication for the use of antibiotics prophylactically is for people who have been in contact with anyone diagnosed as having meningococcal meningitis.

Obviously, antibiotic therapy should never be undertaken lightly. Most antibiotics can have bothersome side effects; a few antibiotics can permanently maim or even kill. The decision to use an antibiotic should always rest with a doctor and should never be part of self-treatment.

The medical community has been made increasingly aware of the drawbacks and dangers — as well as the unnecessary expense — inherent in the overuse and misuse of antibiotic therapy. An article in a March 1974 issue of *JAMA*, which pointed out many of the negative aspects of antibiotic usage discussed in this chapter, called for the establishment in hospitals of more stringent guidelines for the proper use of antibiotics, with peer review as the chief monitoring system (see page 338). CU's medical consultants applaud the suggestion and hope for its early implementation. If the proposals made in the *JAMA* article are carried out, there might be some impact on the prescribing habits of the office practitioner as well as the physician in hospital practice.

Chapter 29

How to stock a medicine cabinet

A FEW SIMPLE, SAFE, AND EFFECTIVE medical supplies, most of them inexpensive, ought to be in any home medicine cabinet. In the following pages CU's medical consultants recommend everything really needed to meet the common medical problems of most families and to cope with the emergencies most frequently encountered in the home. These supplies need be supplemented only if there are special problems, or if additions are recommended by the family physician.

DRUGS TO KEEP ON HAND

Many bathroom medicine cabinets contain a jumble of ancient bottles and plastic containers, some without labels or identifying marks, some holding but one or two mysterious tablets. Periodically, check your medicine cabinet and throw out the accumulation of unidentified or outdated prescription medicines (see page 322). At the same time, make sure you have on hand the seven basic drugs CU's medical consultants recommend for the home medicine cabinet: an analgesic/antipyretic, an antacid, an antidiarrheal remedy, an antipruritic, an antiseptic, a decongestant, and a laxative. *Remember that any drug is potentially dangerous. Therefore all medicines should be stored out of the reach of children.*

ANALGESIC/ANTIPYRETIC (see Chapter 1). Buy the least costly aspirin tablets you can find. (If you or anyone in your family is allergic to aspirin, acetaminophen may be substituted.) In homes where aspirin is used mainly for an occasional headache, menstrual cramps, or the aches and pains caused by a cold, a 100-tablet bottle is the size to buy; for more frequent use, buy a larger size. From time to time, check to be sure the tablets have not begun to crumble excessively — which may happen in high-humidity areas. Sometimes aspirin rectal suppositories may be useful, especially when nausea or vomiting may preclude taking aspirin by mouth.

For children the usual 5-grain aspirin tablet can easily be broken or cut into halves or quarters to obtain the proper dosage, and then crushed. It can be made quite palatable by mixing with applesauce, honey, or jelly.

Parents should think twice before buying children's flavored aspirin. Small children who identify such tablets with candy may be tempted to help themselves. Aspirin in large doses can be fatal. Figures for 1974 show that for children under five about 18 percent of all reported poisoning fatalities were due to ingestion of aspirin or other salicylates. Annual statistics for *ingestion* of aspirin by children less than five years old show that the number of such ingestions have been dropping. In 1974, 5,861 cases were reported, a decrease of about 2,000 from the previous year's total.

So-called tamper-proof caps, required under the Poison Prevention Packaging Act of 1971, are helpful but are certainly not perfect prevention. The directives for administering the act say as much: "Special packaging does not mean packaging that all children under five years of age are unable to open or to obtain a harmful amount within a reasonable time." A child who is above-average in dexterity, persistence, and ingenuity might well open a "tamper-proof" aspirin bottle. Tamper proof or not, precautions must be taken to help prevent ingestion by curious children. A false sense of security could be fatal.

ANTACID (see Chapter 7). Sodium bicarbonate is useful for the treatment of occasional heartburn or other symptoms of simple indigestion — except for those people on a low-sodium diet. If you prefer to use an over-the-counter remedy, read its label carefully; check the list of ingredients to see whether extraneous medication (headache remedies, laxatives, sedatives, etc.) has been added. The closer the product is to a simple antacid, which does nothing more than combat gastric hyperacidity, the better.

ANTIDIARRHEAL REMEDY (see Chapter 8). For diarrhea that may occur from a mild intestinal infection or from a tainted dinner, some people find a kaolin/pectin suspension helpful — even though its efficacy has not yet been proved. For a more protracted case of diarrhea, a physician should be consulted so that a medication of increased potency can be prescribed.

ANTIPRURITIC (see Chapter 13). Ordinary calamine lotion can be used for the relief of mild skin eruptions such as mosquito bites, prickly heat, or poison ivy. A compress of cool tap water may also be helpful. For the relief of severe skin eruptions, compresses of very hot water may prove soothing, but should only be used to treat small areas of skin.

ANTISEPTIC (see Chapter 12). Isopropyl (70 percent) alcohol — usually purchased as rubbing alcohol — is the only antiseptic normally needed in the home. In most cases, minor wounds can be adequately treated just by allowing the wound to bleed a little and washing gently with soap and water. For more protection, swab the skin around the wound with alcohol, but try not to get alcohol in the wound.

DECONGESTANT (see Chapter 2). Phenylephrine hydrochloride solution USP ½ percent may be used as a nasal spray or as nose drops, two or three times a day at most, to reduce the stuffiness of a common cold. This drug deteriorates in storage so buy only ½ ounce at a time. (Use ¼ percent solution for infants and children.) An alternative for some might be an oral decongestant (see page 41).

LAXATIVE (see Chapter 8). If dietary measures do not bring relief from constipation, it is best to have on hand for occasional use a mild laxative such as methylcellulose, psyllium, or dioctyl sodium sulfosuccinate.

HOME FIRST-AID AND SICK-ROOM EQUIPMENT

ADHESIVE BANDAGES. Those with plastic-coated gauze do not stick to a wound. Avoid the tinted medicated type, which may cause an allergic skin reaction.

ROLL BANDAGE, 2 inches wide.

STERILE GAUZE PADS, 4 inches square, separately wrapped.

ADHESIVE TAPE, one small roll 1 or 2 inches wide.

SCISSORS, large enough and sharp enough to cut gauze or cloth.

ELASTIC BANDAGES, about 3 inches wide, for wrapping sprained joints. Be careful not to apply them too tightly.

TWEEZERS, with fine points for removing splinters.

ICE BAG, to minimize bleeding and also to relieve acute pain resulting from injury to joints and muscles. Cold (*not* heat) should be applied immediately following the injury and then intermittently up to twenty-four hours thereafter, using a towel between the skin and the ice bag. After twenty-four hours, mild heat may be beneficial in reducing swelling. Injured joints should be kept relatively immobile to allow torn tendons and muscles to heal.

HOT-WATER BOTTLE OR ELECTRIC HEATING PAD, for mild muscular aches. Extreme care should be taken to avoid burning the skin. Never use a heating pad in conjunction with liniment or any external analgesic; severe blistering may result.

TWO CLINICAL THERMOMETERS, one rectal, one oral. Make sure

the numerical divisions on the thermometers are easy to read.

ENEMA EQUIPMENT. While relatively expensive, prepacked disposable enemas (such as *Fleet*) can be a convenience.

ELECTRIC VAPORIZER, for relief of acute respiratory symptoms (see page 47). A child with croup can often find quick relief in a bathroom steamed up by running the hot water — preferably in the shower — full force.

FIRST-AID MANUAL. The most comprehensive and authoritative of such publications for the general public is the American National Red Cross's *Standard First Aid and Personal Safety*. A copy may be obtained from local chapters for $1.95. This new version of the old *First Aid Textbook* also includes information useful for vacation campers and others who spend much time out in the country or in the woods.

PHONE NUMBER LIST, including both day and night numbers of the family doctor, the nearest poison control center, your pharmacist, the local police or fire department (which often provides emergency services, such as an ambulance or oxygen), and, if available, the volunteer ambulance corps.

SOME ITEMS *NOT* RECOMMENDED

CU's medical consultants believe the following products should be omitted as serving no useful purpose, even though they may be recommended by some authorities or are traditionally included in the medicine cabinet:

ANTISEPTICS such as *Mercurochrome*, tincture of *Merthiolate*, and similar mercury antiseptics; also tincture of iodine. Ordinary rubbing alcohol is the sensible choice of antiseptic (see Chapter 12).

AROMATIC SPIRITS OF AMMONIA, frequently recommended for the treatment of fainting. The only necessary thing to do if someone faints is to place the victim in a horizontal position and await recovery. This usually occurs in a minute or two —

any period of unconsciousness lasting longer than a few minutes warrants medical attention. Do not force any liquids down the throat of an unconscious or semiconscious person; such heroics may result in a near-drowned victim as well.

BORIC ACID SOLUTIONS AND POWDERS. In 1973 Canada prohibited the sale of products containing boric acid or sodium borate to be used as teething preparations or topical applications for infants and children less than three years of age. Canada also requires a warning label on all drugs containing these compounds. CU's medical consultants believe that boric acid solutions and powders offer no medical benefits, and in view of possible toxicity should not be in home medicine cabinets.

COUGH SYRUPS AND ELIXIRS. Any cough that cannot be relieved within a week by steam inhalation, hot drinks, or sucking hard candies should be checked by a physician (see Chapter 3).

OVER-THE-COUNTER BURN OINTMENTS, because they contain antiseptics or anesthetics such as benzocaine, may cause allergic skin reactions in some people. Instead, use ice water or cold running water for the emergency treatment of minor burns (see Chapter 12).

AEROSOL SPRAY PRODUCTS: A WARNING

The pressurized aerosol can is ubiquitous. Household items from oven cleaners and rug shampoos to air fresheners and furniture polishes are packaged in aerosol form. An American family buys, on average, dozens of such products annually. Claims for their convenience are often valid, but the price is high. And by their very nature, aerosol packagings are wasteful of materials used in their production. Most products marketed in aerosol containers are also available in some nonpressurized form, and at much lower cost to the environment and to the consumer.

Over the years there have been reports of death, injury, or

property damage resulting from exploding aerosol containers, usually when the cans were disposed of after final use. But there have been few controlled studies of hazards to human health associated with the actual use of aerosol products. Even so, there have been enough reports of harmful effects to warrant strong suspicion about these products, especially the aerosol spray types.

Products usually need to be specially formulated for aerosol packaging. Standard ingredients must be supplemented by a propellant system to eject the product from the container. Additional solvents, dispersants, and other chemicals must often be included in the reformulation. Some products are expelled as foam, such as shaving cream, or extruded, such as snack food. Others, such as hair spray, are propelled as fine droplets into the air. It is the aerosol sprays that appear to have the greatest potential for hazards in use.

As a result, CU's medical consultants warn against the indiscriminate use of aerosol spray products in the home. Certain decongestant aerosol sprays have already been removed from the market (see Chapter 2), and other aerosol sprays are under investigation. While there may be little cause for concern about the occasional use of an aerosol spray, it is the prolonged and repeated exposure to aerosol sprays that CU's medical consultants consider potentially harmful.

Certain aerosol propellant gases and solvents are flammable, and there have been reports of accidental ignition of various aerosol sprays while in use. The inhalation of other propellant gases has been shown to produce abnormal heart rhythms in laboratory animals, and is thought to be the cause of sudden death of people who have deliberately inhaled the propellant gases. Consequently, CU's medical consultants warn patients who are being treated for heart disease to avoid the use of aerosol spray products.

Some clinical investigators have linked inadvertent inhalation of spray deodorants to a lung disease called sarcoidosis. Experiments with animals chronically exposed to aerosol deodorants have duplicated the lung condition. A chemical type of pneumonia in human beings has been attributed to the use of aerosol sprays. There is some evidence that prolonged use of aerosol sprays can reduce the ability to cough up mucus and to ward off lung infections; CU's medical consultants believe this should be of special concern to people with chronic lung diseases, such as asthma, chronic bronchitis, and emphysema.

The exposed portions of the body are also subject to hazards. The skin may develop irritations from aerosol sprays. Most vulnerable, perhaps, are the eyes; reported injuries range from minor irritation from the chemicals to severe damage from impact of the spray.

If you must use aerosol spray products in the home, we urge you to take precautions:

■ Never use aerosol spray products in a confined area.

■ Keep the spray away from the eyes.

■ Try not to breathe in the spray.

Better yet, CU's medical consultants suggest, avoid unnecessary risks to your health and do not use aerosol sprays in the home. There usually is some other form of the product that costs less — and that may save you more than money.

Chapter 30

How to buy prescription drugs

PRESCRIPTION DRUG SALES in the United States came to about $5 billion in 1972, according to the Council on Economic Priorities. Profits enjoyed by drug manufacturers have been equally impressive. Over the past ten years the drug industry has ranked as one of the two most profitable manufacturing industries in the country (the other is soft drinks).

For many years CU has tried to help consumers avoid contributing unduly to the profitable status of drug companies. CU has advised those who purchase prescription drugs — especially the higher-priced ones — to try to save money by buying, whenever possible, the generic form of the drug, which may cost less than the brand-name version of the product. Since prices vary from pharmacy to pharmacy, CU has also urged consumers who are not confronted with a medical emergency to take the time to comparison shop before having a prescription filled.

Indeed, numerous surveys have repeatedly documented the wide disparity in pricing of prescription drugs — and the value of comparison shopping. For example, CU made a prescription shopping test in the New York metropolitan area a few years ago. Given a prescription for thirty capsules of tetracycline, the generic name for a commonly used broad-spectrum anti-

314

biotic (see Chapter 28), CU shoppers went to sixty drugstores. The prices they had to pay ranged from 79¢ all the way to $7.45. The results of CU's test shopping have been confirmed by other agencies — governmental, trade, and private — that have undertaken similar drug price surveys.

The American Medical Association (AMA) made a study several years ago in the Chicago area. AMA shoppers filled 686 prescriptions for seven drugs at 185 drugstores. One of the drugs bought was meprobamate, marketed as Miltown by Wallace, as Equanil by Wyeth, and by generic name by other companies. In all, 159 prescriptions for this drug were filled, each calling for twenty-five tablets containing 0.4 grams per tablet. Forty-nine pharmacies filled prescriptions calling for Miltown at prices ranging from $1.63 to $4.95. Sixty-two prescriptions calling for the same amount of Equanil were filled at prices ranging from $1.72 to $4.05. Prescriptions calling only for meprobamate, without specifying a brand name, were filled by forty-eight pharmacies. Half of them supplied either Miltown or Equanil, at prices ranging from $1.25 to $4.40. The other half provided tablets not identifiable by brand name, at prices ranging from $1.25 to $4. (Startling variations were also found in the prices charged for the other drugs in the AMA survey.)

Until recently, few consumers had easy access to price information about prescription drugs. The laws and regulations of many states prohibited the advertising of prescription drug prices. In other states pharmaceutical trade groups and state boards of pharmacy tended to pressure stores not to post prices or advertise prescription costs. To some extent, these practices were challenged in court cases which upheld the right of several large drug chains to make price information public. Accelerating the process of informing the public were federal anti-inflation measures in 1972, which required pharmacies to compile data about pricing and to make the information available to customers who requested it.

Several states ultimately forced the issue. New York State pharmacists have been required since January 1, 1974, to post prominently the names and prices of the 150 most frequently prescribed drugs. (Boston has enforced such regulations since 1971.) As of this writing, California, Connecticut, Maryland, Michigan, Minnesota, Nevada, New Hampshire, Texas, and Vermont also require posting some prescription drug prices.

The Food and Drug Administration (FDA) intervened toward the close of 1973 to help standardize the pricing information to be given to consumers. Beginning in January 1976, the agency has prescribed the format to be used for posting and advertising of prescription drug prices. Through its regulations, the FDA hopes to ensure a uniform national system which will provide consumers "with information needed to make meaningful price comparisons."

CU reminds consumers that until states require pharmacies to post the prices of *all* drugs, it may pay to check on the cost of a prescription before it is filled, and then compare the price at another pharmacy.

Even if all states were to require full disclosure of prescription drug prices, there would still be limits to the efficacy of comparison shopping for drugs. Because of the nature of the drug industry, and the effect of patent laws, certain drugs dominate the United States market. And in some instances, the cooperation of your physician and pharmacist will be necessary. The following review of the process by which new prescription drugs are marketed may, to some extent, help consumers avoid overspending for medications.

During the period in which a new drug is undergoing clinical investigation, it is given its *generic* name by the United States Adopted Names Council (a semiofficial organization sponsored by the AMA, the United States Pharmacopeial Convention, and the American Pharmaceutical Association). The generic name is usually a simplified word version of the chemical formulation. Once the FDA has declared the drug to be both safe and effective, and therefore ready for marketing, the pharmaceutical firm decides on a *brand* name for its new product; this name is then registered as a trademark. From the manufacturer's point of view, the ideal brand name is one that will stick tenaciously in the memory of prescribing physicians.

Patent rights, ordinarily lasting for seventeen years, protect the new drug from duplication by rival firms. During that period, the company holding the patent enjoys exclusive rights to production and sales — unless it decides to license, for a fee, other firms to market the drug. During the life of the patent, a prescription written for the new drug by its generic name may cost just as much as one written by its brand name. For example, diazepam — better known by its brand name, Valium — was developed by a Swiss-based firm, Hoffman-La Roche, the world's largest drug company, which has about two-fifths of its sales in the United States market. Since other firms are excluded from production, prescriptions written for diazepam can be filled only with Valium as long as the patent holds.

When a patent expires, other firms may then manufacture the drug. The patent holder, however, retains the right to the original brand name. Competing companies must invent their own brand names, or market the product under its generic name. The price of the original brand-name drug may fall; the cut in price is affected by the number of competing products, market demand, and promotion to physicians. Despite advertising to physicians and efforts of rival detail men (see Chapter 26), the original drug firm retains a considerable advantage even after the patent rights expire, because the medical profession has for so long equated the product with the original brand name. To this day, Abbott Laboratories enjoys large profits from the sale of Nembutal (a barbiturate-type sleeping medication with the generic name pentobarbital), despite the expiration of patent rights, and despite the fact that many smaller companies sell their versions of pentobarbital for a fraction of the price charged for Nembutal. Doctors who specify a brand name in a prescription in effect compel their patients to enrich the manufacturer of that brand-name drug.

Brand-name prescription drugs often cost five to ten times more than their generic counterparts — and sometimes even up to thirty times more. Understandably, the drug industry has not been enthusiastic about the efforts of CU and other consumer organizations and of legislators who advocate prescription by generic name. Industry spokesmen often question the quality of generic drugs. CU's medical consultants do not believe that the price of a medicine is a reliable guide to its quality.

The quality of prescription drugs marketed in the United States is monitored by the FDA through two large centers for drug analysis. The National Center for Antibiotics in Washington, D.C., is responsible for certifying the potency, purity, and stability of every antibiotic, batch by batch, prior to marketing. The National Center for Drug Analysis in St. Louis has since 1970 completed a study of nineteen other classes of drugs, including, among others, adrenocorticosteroids, major and minor tranquilizers, urinary antibacterial agents, central nervous system depressants, antithyroid agents, cardiac drugs, anticoagulants, and oral contraceptives. The study has been extended to cover every known manufacturer of the top fifteen most important drug classes.

These efforts on the part of the FDA led Dr. Henry E. Simmons, then head of its Bureau of Drugs, to state in 1972: "On the basis of the data we have accrued to date we cannot conclude there is a significant difference in quality between the generic and brand-name product tested." Both large and small companies have been involved in lapses in quality control.

Proponents of brand-name drugs have also questioned the therapeutic equivalence of brand-name and generic products.

An important factor in the determination of therapeutic equivalence is the bioavailability of a drug. In the case of a drug taken orally, this represents the amount of active medication absorbed from the intestine into the bloodstream, thus making the drug available to perform its function. Bioavailability can be evaluated by analyzing the blood of patients who have ingested a drug. In such fashion, blood levels of chemically identical drugs can be compared and, if found similar, therapeutic equivalence may be presumed. Differences in bioavailability have been attributed to variations in the formulation of products. Drug companies may use a variety of inert ingredients, known to the trade as stabilizers, binders, and so forth, in the manufacturing process. These ingredients may or may not affect absorption of a drug (and thus its bioavailability).

It is the United States Pharmacopeia (USP) — see page 368 — that sets the standards for laboratory testing of drugs to ensure quality and purity. One test related to the question of bioavailability is that for dissolution — how quickly the active ingredient in, say, a tablet being tested passes into solution. In contrast to tests for disintegration — how quickly the tablet breaks up into smaller particles of specified size — performance in dissolution tests does correlate with bioavailability. Beginning in 1970, dissolution time specifications have been required by the USP for several drug classes including digoxin (a commonly used heart drug), hydrochlorothiazide (a diuretic), meprobamate (a tranquilizer), phenylbutazone (an anti-inflammatory drug), prednisone (a cortisone analogue), sulfisoxazole and nitrofurantoin (urinary antibiotics), and tolbutamide (an oral hypoglycemic). CU's medical consultants endorse the addition of dissolution time tests to USP standards for these drugs. The tightening of standards helps insure the therapeutic equivalence of chemically identical drugs made by different manufacturers, as well as different batches of a drug made by the same firm. CU's medical consultants urge the addition of more drugs to the list, so that the chances of differences in bioavailability will be narrowed even further.

The actual number of instances in which differences in bioavailability have been demonstrated are relatively small — a fraction of the prescription drug market. With the current FDA and USP controls in operation, defective products and differences in bioavailability are less likely to go undetected.

The generic versus brand name controversy is part of a long struggle between consumer groups and the drug industry to lower drug costs without sacrificing quality. CU believes that the use of brand names for drugs should be completely eliminated, and that all drugs should be designated only by generic name. (A bill to this effect was introduced in the Senate in October 1973 by Senator Gaylord Nelson of Wisconisn.) If the belief persists that price is indicative of quality — or if the last detail man's sales pitch casts a spell — a physician could still specify a particular manufacturer's more costly version. But when no manufacturer is singled out on the prescription blank, the mandatory use of the generic name should help the consumer to purchase the least expensive of several equivalent products on the pharmacist's shelves.

In addition to savings for the consumer, the elimination of brand names for prescription drugs might also benefit some doctors — and ultimately their patients. The FDA has estimated that about seven hundred drugs are marketed under about twenty thousand brand names — which means an average of thirty different names for each of the prescription drugs. The profusion of brand names inevitably creates confusion for many busy physicians. The tale has been told of a hapless physician who prescribed Lederle's Achromycin for a patient's respiratory infection. When the patient showed no improvement, the doctor then prescribed, also to no avail, Squibb's Sumycin, followed by Bristol's Tetrex, little realizing that these were all brand names for the same drug, tetracycline. If CU's proposal for the mandatory use of generic names were fully implemented, there would be less reason to repeat such stories.

Physicians may have increased incentive to prescribe generically if a program announced by the Secretary of Health, Education, and Welfare (HEW) in December 1973 becomes effective. HEW proposed to limit reimbursement for any drug under Medicare and Medicaid "to the lowest cost at which the drug is generally available unless there is a demonstrated difference in therapeutic effect."

Even with the exclusive use of generic names for prescription drugs, much would still depend on the pharmacist, as well as on the commitment of the consumer to comparison shopping. For example, there are no cost benefits for the patient who brings a prescription for generic chlorpheniramine (an antihistamine) to a pharmacist who stocks only Schering's brand, Chlor-Trimeton. The pharmacist, while still forbidden in many states to substitute a generic drug for a prescribed brand name, may legally sell a higher-priced brand-name product if a generic is specified. Therefore a consumer whose physician has written a generic prescription must still check prices at a few pharmacies in order to obtain the lowest price.

Here are some additional suggestions about prescription drugs from CU's medical consultants:

■ Discuss with your physician the correct dosage and time for taking a prescribed drug. Ask that the prescription state that these medication instructions be included on the drug label. Advice to "Take as directed" is not much help if you forget the doctor's instructions — or never clearly understood them in the first place.

■ For drugs that are taken regularly, check to see if you can save money by buying as large a quantity as will stay fresh at the rate you use them (ask your pharmacist).

■ If your state does not already have such a requirement, ask your physician to direct the pharmacist to include on each prescription drug label the name of the drug, its strength, the amount (number of tablets, ounces, etc.), and the expiration date (the date after which the medication is no longer sure to be fully effective, or may be harmful). With this information available to you, leftover portions of some prescriptions could still be used if the family physician prescribes the same medication again. Do not, however, use such leftovers until you have checked with your doctor and confirmed that they are the correct medicine in the proper dosage. Such information on the label could also be life-saving should anyone take an overdose of a medication.

▪ Discard all prescriptions by their expiration date.

Some consumers may have no choice about where to fill a prescription — especially in an emergency situation. Even for those who can shop around, it may be best to stick with a single pharmacy once comparison pricing has shown the charges to be consistently reasonable. The price differential between a neighborhood drugstore and the pharmacy in a large cutrate drugstore or in a department store may be less important than the service extras the local pharmacy may offer. The neighborhood pharmacist usually keeps records of your purchases of prescription medications. Such records can be important in preventing or tracing allergic reactions to drugs; they can also help avoid the dispensing of incompatible drugs. For those who can afford the markup, such personal service, plus home delivery, and possible assistance in emergencies may be worth the extra money involved.

Chapter 31

How to look for a family doctor

THERE IS NO DOUBT that a large number of people are seriously concerned about current medical practices. Much of this concern legitimately focuses on the economics of medicine — the rising cost of medical services, of hospital care, and of drugs. But the discontent also has less concrete causes. Patients complain that doctors are not as friendly as they used to be; they are cold, callous; they shift patients back and forth from one doctor to another; they are never there when you want them; and so on.

Such feelings stem from a basic disruption in the traditional relationship between family doctors and their patients, a disruption that in turn is an outgrowth of profound change throughout our society.

Since the turn of the century the United States has shifted from a predominantly rural or semirural society to a predominantly urban and suburban society. Our grandparents usually had no trouble choosing a doctor — there was only one in town. Today, in most communities, there is such a bewildering variety of family doctors and specialists within reasonable reach that many families put off selecting a physician until illness forces a hurried choice. Under such circumstances, that choice may not always be the best one.

The position of a doctor in relation to patients and their care has also changed. For patients, most medical care used to be a matter of seeing one doctor. Now the family doctor is at the head of a team which changes with the demands of the patients' illnesses. A physician specializes to such a degree that for an illness of some complexity three or four specialists quite legitimately may be needed to help in diagnosis or treatment. And, of course, there are many paramedical health professionals (nurses, laboratory technicians, etc.) who provide necessary services to patients.

This century has seen a drastic shift even in the kinds of diseases that are prevalent. With the development of immunization procedures and antibiotics, epidemic infectious diseases have largely been controlled. This in turn has increased life expectancy; as more of us live longer, the incidence of chronic physical and mental illness mounts. As a result, more and more people are in need of long-term medical supervision.

The changes in how we live and the ills that beset us have only intensified the need for a family medical adviser. In line with the common human tendency to hark back to a golden age, many of us recall nostalgically the family doctor of a generation or two ago, who so often was a friend and adviser. In those days, the family doctor was always a general practitioner and, for all practical purposes, general practitioner and family doctor were synonymous.

Today there is a great deal of puzzlement over the "disappearance" of the old-time family doctor. But if we define a family doctor as one who acts as an all-around medical adviser for the family, treats many ailments personally, and calls in help for a difficult problem, such a doctor really has not disappeared at all. The confusion arises because of the continued identification of the family doctor with the general practitioner. Many people still limit themselves to general practitioners when they seek a family doctor. To understand why this course of action so often brings disappointment, we need to note what has happened within the medical profession in recent decades — and, to a large degree, is continuing to happen. Before World War II close to two-thirds of all practicing physicians were general practitioners; today slightly more than one-third are, according to figures from the American Medical Association (AMA).

Certainly, one factor contributing to the decrease in the number of family doctors was the change in the basic structure of American medicine with the formation of medical specialty boards. The first one was established in ophthalmology in 1917. Today there are twenty-two such groups, all members of the American Board of Medical Specialties. Each of these boards is responsible for the establishment of training requirements, other qualifications, and the administration of certifying examinations in a particular specialty area. A physician who passes the American Board examination within a specialty area becomes *board-certified*, and is known as a diplomate of that board. Many physicians who are *board-eligible* by virtue of their training have not taken the qualifying examinations.

In many of the twenty-two board specialties, a doctor may also be a member of a "college," an honorary body whose main concern is continuing medical education within the specialty. Once certain qualifications have been met, the physician may be elected a fellow of the college. Such organizations include, for example, the American College of Obstetrics and Gynecology, the American Academy of Pediatrics, the American College of Physicians, or the American College of Surgeons. Thus such initials as FACOG, FAAP, FACP, or FACS after a physician's MD* show that the physician is a fellow of a

* Some doctors use the initials PC following the MD. The initials PC do not in any way signify professional qualification or achievement. They stand for professional corporation; the laws of many states now permit doctors to incorporate.

particular college, and very probably a diplomate in that specialty. A comprehensive listing of all diplomates of the various specialty boards is published in the *Directory of Medical Specialists,* available in some libraries.

American Board certification usually means that the physician's practice is restricted to the specialty. And, from the doctor's point of view, American Board certification is becoming increasingly important. Most specialists who want hospital affiliations and prestige, from which referrals and important sources of income are derived, usually need to be board-certified. Board certification is also important to specialists because they are paid higher fees by insurance companies and the like.

Prospective patients should be forewarned that any physician can legally practice surgical or medical specialties without the specialized training that board certification represents. Therefore, the initials such as those just identified afford some reassurance that a physician is qualified in a specialty. Such identification can be quite helpful to the prospective patient who should not assume that every hospital actually screens a specialist's qualifications. While it is unlikely that a reputable hospital would allow an unqualified practitioner to apply complex medical or surgical techniques, this may not be universally true.

During the first quarter of this century the relatively small amount of medical knowledge, and the slow rate of change in that knowledge, made general medical practice a logical and reasonable professional career. Then began the scientific advances that have escalated in the last twenty years. Because most doctors cannot master the entire field of medicine, they have tended to concentrate on smaller and smaller segments. Even in the area of surgery the multiplicity of new procedures is forcing surgeons toward further specialization.

Medical schools have reinforced the impetus toward specialization. Departments of medicine and surgery are subdivided into sections for each of the subspecialty areas. Because of the complexity of modern diagnosis, treatment, and rehabilitation, it takes specialists to teach each subject. Specialization therefore has its roots in teaching institutions and, as a consequence, medical students frequently develop strong interests in a specialty area.

For today's doctor, hospitals are both workshops and centers for continuing education in the specialty area. At the hospital a physician's medical knowledge is reinforced and expanded through conferences, discussions, and association with colleagues, as well as experience with patients. Particularly during rounds in teaching hospitals (see page 340), the physicians and house staff share opinions, knowledge, and experience.

Because continuing education is so crucial to the professional standing of many doctors, positions on the staff of a teaching hospital are sought after. And such hospitals, in order to maintain their character and reputation, usually insist that a prospective staff member be well qualified. Standards at any hospital are most likely to remain high when the medical and surgical subspecialties are well represented.

Some effort is being made within the medical profession to offset the tide of specialization. The American Academy of Family Physicians (AAFP) is the most widely known of the organizations dedicated to the revitalization of general practice. The AAFP requirements for membership make mandatory one of the following: three years of approved graduate training, two years of graduate training plus two years of general practice, or one year of graduate training plus three years of general practice during which the applicant must complete 150 hours of approved education. After being accepted for membership, all who wish to continue as active members are then required to complete 150 hours of accredited postgraduate study every three years. There are more than thirty thousand members, plus fifty-four hundred additional student affiliates. Osteopathic physicians (see page 331) are also eligible for membership.

In 1970, medicine appeared to have come full circle when the specialty of generalists, "family practice," received board certification status and the American Board of Family Practice conducted its first certifying examination. By the end of 1975, there were 7,015 physicians certified in family practice. More than three-quarters of these physicians are also members of the AAFP.

In addition, state and local medical societies have set up sections on general practice, and many medical schools have established professorships and departments of family practice — all dedicated to revitalizing the role of the family physician. It appears likely that these efforts may offset to some extent the trend to specialization. Undoubtedly, family practice will occupy an increasingly important place in medicine in the United States. While the new specialty grows, many patients turn to the internist for primary medical care.

An internist is a physician with postgraduate training in internal medicine — that is, in all areas of medicine except surgical, obstetric, and pediatric practice. By the end of 1975, 30,372 diplomates were certified by the American Board of Internal Medicine. In addition, there are thousands of board-eligible physicians who are well-qualified internists.

Within the broad field of internal medicine there are subspecialty areas, each of which has its own subspecialty board. These areas include allergy, cardiology, endocrinology, gastroenterology, hematology, nephrology, oncology, pulmonary disease, and rheumatology.

Whether certified or eligible, the internists' training and expertise in internal medicine should make them more capable of dealing with heart and kidney disease, diabetes, and arthritis, as well as disorders affecting the blood and endocrine systems. Since more than half of the illnesses they deal with in routine office practice are psychogenic, they can help with this aspect of patient treatment. Their training should also increase their interest in the occupational and social aspects of disease. Because of this broad training and interest, internists are usually well qualified to serve as family medical advisers and consultants. They can take care of most common disorders themselves, but refer patients to other specialists when a disorder requires more specialized care.

Medical care from a board-certified or board-eligible internist, or from an up-to-date general practitioner — one certified in family practice or an AAFP member — is not, of course, automatically assured to be of the highest quality. But it does greatly increase the chances.

In several states such chances are enhanced somewhat by specific requirements physicians must meet in order to remain in good standing in their profession. Although all doctors must be licensed by their respective state boards of medical examiners, in most states renewal of licenses is a mere formality. Only New Mexico, as of this writing, makes renewal of the license to practice medicine contingent upon the completion of a prescribed amount of accredited postgraduate study in medicine.

Most state and county medical societies have been slow to support mandatory postgraduate education in medicine. In fourteen states medical societies have gone on record endorsing the principle of requiring continuing medical education as a condition of membership renewal. However, as of this writing, only four state medical societies — Arizona, New Jersey, Oregon (which pioneered the concept), and Pennsylvania — actually have such a procedure in operation. California's medical society has a unique program with even more stringent standards than the typical mandatory requirement of 150 hours of postgraduate study over a three-year period — but it is voluntary.

The medical establishment has made its most widespread attempt to promote professional competence through voluntary self-assessment programs. Since 1968, the American College of Physicians (ACP) has encouraged all physicians who consider themselves internists to take what amounts to an open-book examination consisting of about 700 questions. Starting with the second self-assessment program in 1971, physicians who give their consent permit the ACP to score their examinations and to group the results. In this way gaps in knowledge are made more apparent to agencies planning programs of continuing medical education.

The various specialty boards — with one exception — have not used periodic reexamination as a means of insuring continued high levels of professionalism. At the present time only one specialty, family practice, has built into its method of operation the requirement that reexamination at regular intervals is needed for continued certification. The first certifying examination for family practice was held in 1970. In 1976 those who qualified in 1970 may once again qualify for certification by taking a second examination as part of an overall review of continued eligibility for certification in family practice. None of the other specialty boards has as yet followed suit, although since 1971 those who took tests leading to American Board certification in internal medicine have been asked to acknowledge the possibility that they might be retested at some future date. And only family practice has, in effect, done away with the possibility of remaining board-eligible but not board-certified. CU believes that more should be done by the other medical specialty boards to encourage board-eligible physicians to prepare for and take the examinations leading to certification.

As of 1974 the ACP will associate self-assessment with recertification. On a strictly voluntary basis, board-certified internists who join in the third self-assessment offered by the ACP may take a recertification examination prepared in conjunction with the American Board of Internal Medicine. Thus internists who participate in both aspects of the program expose themselves not only to the perils of self-knowledge, but also to the test of meeting current standards of competence.

CU endorses the efforts of various medical societies and of state boards of medical examiners to require postgraduate study for practicing physicians. Until better mechanisms are devised to enhance the quality of the medical professional, CU believes that the most effective way to cull the incompetent is periodic, mandatory examination.

Another category of health professional available for family medical care is the osteopathic physician. Osteopathy is becoming increasingly recognized by organized medicine, both on national and state levels. Graduates of schools of osteopathy, of which there are currently ten in the United States, are given a postgraduate education not dissimilar in many respects to that offered by medical schools. There are currently about 15,500 osteopathic physicians, approximately 75 percent of whom are in family practice. As with MDs, doctors of osteopathy (DOs) may become certified in the various specialties by taking qualifying examinations administered by one of the American Osteopathic Boards. Most of the twenty-two boards of medical specialties also now permit osteopaths to qualify for certification examinations; prominent exceptions are the American Board of Surgery and several surgically related boards. In 1968 the AMA made osteopaths eligible for membership; as of mid-1973, 125 DOs had joined.

The American Osteopathic Association claims that osteopathic medicine "goes beyond general medicine in its distinctive recognition of the function of the musculoskeletal system in health and disease." CU's medical consultants, as MDs, do not agree with the following statement of the American Osteopathic Association: "Diagnostic and therapeutic methods applied to [the musculoskeletal] system make osteopathic medicine today's most comprehensive and complete approach to man's health problems."

Osteopaths are *not* to be confused with chiropractors, who are, in the opinion of CU's medical consultants, no substitute for medical professionals. Chiropractic is based upon unscientific and unproved methods of treatment.

Even if you would like to confine your search for a family doctor to an internist, you may not be able to locate one who can take on new patients. In that case, you may find the family medical adviser you are seeking in a general practitioner — one with a limited practice who does not deliver babies or perform major surgery. Such physicians have developed a medical practice that parallels in many ways the work of the internist.

The category of ideal family doctor, therefore, in addition to the internist, includes the general practitioner who neither performs major surgery nor practices obstetrics and who is on the staff of an accredited hospital (see Chapter 32). Accredited hospitals keep fairly close tabs on the competence of the physicians on their staffs.

How do you set out to find a family doctor? If you are moving to a new location, the simplest way is to ask your present physician to recommend one. Your physician may be acquainted with doctors in your new area, or may be able to verify for you the qualifications of possible family doctors. Otherwise, after you have moved, check with the nearest accredited hospital. Ask the hospital for a list of internists or general practitioners who are on its staff as attending physicians. If a medical school is situated near your new hometown, a telephone inquiry may produce the names of internists or qualified family doctors on the faculty who practice in your community. The county medical society may also be helpful in providing you with the names of physicians — both internists and general practitioners — in your immediate vicinity. A friend or relative, whose judgment you respect and who knows your likes and dislikes, may often prove to be a valuable lead to a new family doctor.

With a list of qualified candidates, you can make a survey to find one who seems to suit your family as a medical adviser. It would make sense to start with those whose offices are closest to where you live, for convenience as well as prompt care in an emergency. Let the doctor know that you are selecting a family physician, and do not hesitate to inquire about hospital affiliations, attitude toward home calls, and any other questions that concern you. Be sure to inquire about fees. Some doctors bill once a month, some after each visit; others may ask for a deposit in advance of treatment. Most doctors itemize bills on request. (Once having chosen the key physician, you can then expect assistance in selecting specialists, as the need arises.)

No matter what process you have used, the physician you select could in the long run turn out to be unacceptable. Personalities may clash, you may not like an office nurse, or you may object to long interludes in a waiting room. The doctor may indulge in "scare tactics" or may be too rushed to discuss details of your case with you. The office may be so poorly organized that messages do not get through. Under these circumstances, it might be best to look around for another doctor.

On the other hand, the chronic doctor shopper rarely benefits from an apparently endless search for the ideal doctor. The patient who drifts from physician to physician in search of a nonexistent remedy or that perfect bedside manner may be the greater loser than the patient who endures one or two uncomfortable encounters with the office bureaucracy or an isolated brusque moment with the doctor.

If a dire emergency develops and no physician can be reached, the quickest source of help in any urban or suburban community is the local police or fire department. Your community might have a volunteer ambulance corps which provides emergency transportation to a hospital. If more time is available and the emergency is not so pressing, call the county medical society, night or day; most county medical societies maintain a roster of physicians who are available to make home calls. Also, remember that most hospitals maintain emergency facilities, available to the public, which are staffed around the clock.

The internist or family doctor you select may be a member of a private group practice. In one type of group practice, several different specialists (for example, an internist, an obstetrician, a pediatrician, and a surgeon) pool their talents and their expensive office equipment, but charge patients on a fee-for-service basis. This arrangement may provide patients with both technical competence and integrated medical care. In many group practices of this type, there are physicians with the competence and the training of internists who are able to serve as family doctors. In another type of group practice, several doctors engaged in the practice of a specialty (for example, internal medicine or pediatrics) work together under one roof and share facilities.

The disadvantages of selecting a doctor in group practice include the possibility of not achieving a permanent relationship with one doctor in particular and the chance that you might be shunted to another doctor within the group. These disadvantages may be outweighed by somewhat lower charges, assurance of treatment by competent physicians should your own doctor in the group be unavailable, and easy access by these doctors to your medical records.

Check also to see if there is a prepaid comprehensive medical service plan in your area, which could provide the services of a qualified internist or family doctor. For some patients, such a facility might save money. Known as HMOs (health maintenance organizations), these plans offer subscribers a variety of medical services for a fixed monthly fee paid in advance. There are usually no separate charges for any type of medical care provided under such plans. Most of these plans are associated with the Group Health Association of America, 1717 Massachusetts Avenue, N.W., Washington, D.C. 20036.

Readers in rural and semirural communities may find the advice offered here difficult or impossible to follow. Many outlying hospitals do not maintain the high standards that they ought to, and more than three-fourths of rural doctors are general practitioners whose training and competence are difficult if not impossible for prospective patients to evaluate.

The ideal solution in such cases cannot be found on an individual basis. A community guarantee of an adequate income to an internist who has just completed training would help by leveling out the economic disparity between city and rural areas. But it is not easy for the local citizens, even in a relatively populous rural area, to provide a combination of better medical facilities (including a hospital) and cultural, professional, and financial opportunities. Yet that seems to be what it takes to attract and hold qualified doctors and their families.

A partial solution to the medical needs of those who live in sparsely settled areas may be found by organizing, into a regional association, all the voluntary nonprofit hospitals located in and near these areas, assisted, where possible, by the nearest medical school.

The answer to how to choose a dentist is in many ways similar to the suggestions already given for the selection of a doctor. If you are moving, ask your present dentist for a recommendation. Consult county and local dental societies or, where possible, the faculty of a nearby dental college. Check with friends or relatives. And don't forget the valuable resource you now have, your new family doctor, who may be able to recommend a competent dentist.

Chapter 32

What makes
a good hospital

SINCE CU'S METHOD for choosing a family doctor (see Chapter 31) often calls for starting at a nearby accredited hospital, it is necessary to know something about what makes one hospital better than another. Moreover, when the need for hospitalization arises, patients are sometimes offered a choice from among the hospitals with which their doctors are affiliated. For both reasons, consumers ought to have at least some idea of how to judge a hospital. There are three main questions to ask.

1. IS THE HOSPITAL ACCREDITED? The first question is whether the hospital is accredited by the Joint Commission on Accreditation of Hospitals (JCAH). Such accreditation cannot guarantee that a hospital is first-rate, but it can help safeguard against substandard medical care and a hazardous physical plant.

There is no legal requirement that a hospital or any other type of health-care facility be accredited. But the fact that a facility is accredited by the JCAH indicates that it has voluntarily met established standards for its operation and for the delivery of care and services.

The JCAH has four member organizations — the American College of Physicians, the American College of Surgeons, the American Hospital Association, and the American Medical

Association (AMA) — which provide the main financial support for all JCAH accreditation programs. The JCAH also derives income from fees for the hospital surveys it conducts (see below) and from grants. In addition to the Hospital Accreditation Program, the JCAH operates programs for the accreditation of long-term care facilities, psychiatric facilities, and facilities for the mentally retarded.

About two-thirds of the 7,200 general hospitals in the United States are accredited. If a hospital wants to be accredited, it must conform to a set of published standards in every aspect of its operation. The first step is for the hospital to submit an application. After a detailed questionnaire has been completed, the hospital receives an on-site survey by a team composed of a physician and either a hospital administrator or a registered nurse (or all three).

The JCAH survey team makes an extensive examination of the hospital. They ascertain whether the physical plant is properly maintained to meet safety requirements. They verify the ownership of the hospital to determine who is ultimately responsible for the facility's performance. The team checks the bylaws of the hospital, and then decides whether the medical staff follows the bylaws. During the survey the team seeks to determine whether the medical staff is functioning effectively and whether its performance is of the quality necessary to deliver good care.

Particular emphasis is placed on the adequacy and comprehensiveness of medical records, and on a review of medical staff organization. The team meets with members of the hospital staff and examines patient records and the minutes of staff and committee meetings. They inquire into the way privileges are granted and delineated.

The hospital's provisions for monitoring its own performance and its procedures for self-evaluation are also studied by the survey team. The quality of medical care can be judged from the completeness of patients' medical charts, the frequency with which mortality review committees meet, and the details covered in these meetings. The survey team examines the records of peer review committees, organized to determine inconsistencies and deficiencies in the management of patients and to guard against the abuse of hospital privileges, as well as the records of staff utilization committees, which determine whether available bed space is being used efficiently.

The tissue committee, composed of representatives from the departments of surgery and pathology, may turn the spotlight on unnecessary surgery. The pathologist reports to this committee on all the normal tissue removed each month. A surgeon found to have repeatedly removed normal tissue may be called before the committee to explain why. A surgeon whose record does not improve might lose some or all staff privileges.

In checking each service and department, the survey team evaluates the hospital's documented evidence that it is conforming to JCAH standards. The evaluation includes not only the medical records department, but also the laboratories, the X-ray, nursing, and dietary services, the departments of anesthesiology and — if the hospital has them — the departments of physical medicine, pharmacy, medical social services, and emergency services.

When the on-site survey is completed, the team submits its report and recommendations to the JCAH Hospital Accreditation Program. After an overall review, the report and recommendations are sent to the Accreditation Committee of the JCAH's Board of Commissioners. The hospital may receive one of three ratings: two-year accreditation, one-year accreditation, or no accreditation. The decision is communicated to the hospital, together with recommendations for improvement. In 1975 the JCAH surveyed 2,502 hospitals; of these, 72 percent received two-year accreditation, 25 percent received one-year accreditation, and 3 percent were denied accreditation.

Hospitals given accreditation usually display their certificate in the lobby. But if you are uncertain whether a hospital is accredited, you can find out by asking the hospital's administrators or by writing to the Office of Public Information of the Joint Commission on Accreditation of Hospitals, 875 North Michigan Avenue, Chicago, Illinois 60611. Since the Commission's program is fully voluntary, the fact that a hospital is not accredited may simply mean that it has not sought accreditation. But unless you have good reason to do otherwise, you should avoid, if possible, any nonaccredited hospital.

Recently the JCAH has given the consumer of hospital services the opportunity to play a role in the accreditation process. Individuals and representatives of interested groups are now able to request a hearing before the on-site team surveying a hospital for accreditation. The testimony heard at these public information interviews is taken into account, according to the JCAH, both by the survey team and later by the home office when the survey report is evaluated and the accreditation decision made.

The JCAH reports that very few individuals or consumer groups have as yet taken advantage of the provision for a formal hearing before an on-site survey team. Consumers who wish to make more use of the opportunity are being assisted by such organizations as the Consumer Commission on the Accreditation of Health Services (CCAHS), based in New York City. The CCAHS has volunteered to make arrangements, on request, for a public information interview at hospitals in the New York City area. According to JCAH policies ratified in August 1972, a hospital is required to reveal the date of an impending survey, when requested in writing to do so. The hospital is usually advised of the precise date of the survey about six weeks before the visit. The hospital and the JCAH team, if requested in writing, must hold a public information interview at the time of the survey. The CCAHS reports that several major hospitals have made public the JCAH survey results and have also invited consumers to accompany the JCAH survey teams on their inspection tours.

A consumer who is dissatisfied with an accredited hospital need no longer rely solely on a hearing before the JCAH survey team to register a serious objection. Under 1972 amendments to Social Security legislation the Department of Health, Education, and Welfare (HEW) is required to investigate any "substantial allegation" that a hospital receiving funds under Medicare is not complying with prescribed standards of safety and health.

If investigation reveals that a hospital is indeed violating federal standards, Medicare funds may be withheld from the hospital. A consumer who wishes to make a "substantial allegation" should first become familiar with the Medicare standards (copies may be examined at a district Social Security office) and then address the specific complaint to: Social Security Administration, Director of the Bureau of Health Insurance, 640 Security Boulevard, Baltimore, Maryland 21235. CU advises consumers to send copies of such letters to the JCAH, the hospital licensure agency of the state, the Secretary of HEW, and to their senators and representatives.

2. IS IT A "TEACHING" HOSPITAL? One can go beyond the basic question of accreditation in judging the quality and capabilities of a hospital by asking the second question: Does it have a formal program for the training of medical personnel? The higher the level of such teaching, the higher the level of medical services the hospital is likely to provide. The best indicator of a good teaching program is affiliation with a medical school. Hospitals with such affiliation are likely to have available as needed the services of qualified family doctors and specialists in all fields; they often have full-time staff physicians in charge of key departments; and they attract many of the best young physicians who want residency training in the specialties. Such

an environment is also likely to bring out the best in the doctors affiliated with the hospital.

As of 1975, there were 1,168 United States hospitals with some type of formal affiliation with a medical school. Of the 1,168 affiliated hospitals, 401 are also members of the Council of Teaching Hospitals of the Association of American Medical Colleges. To qualify, the 401 institutions, all voluntary hospitals (see page 342), must have residency programs in at least four fields (including two of six major fields: family practice, internal medicine, obstetrics/gynecology, pediatrics, psychiatry, and surgery). Because the country's 116 schools of medicine and affiliated hospitals are not distributed evenly, not all consumers have easy access to a hospital affiliated with a medical school. But somewhat similar benefits can be obtained from a hospital approved for residency training in the specialty fields by the AMA Council on Medical Education. To inquire about medical school affiliation of hospitals in your area write to the Office of Public Affairs, American Hospital Association, 840 North Lake Shore Drive, Chicago, Illinois 60611.

Lacking a hospital affiliated with a medical school, or one approved for residency training, you can next consider a hospital that trains house staff or nurses. Because of the continuing shortage of hospital personnel, however, there have been abuses in both house staff and nursing programs in some hospitals. For example, hospitals have been known to permit student nurses to take full charge of a group of patients, especially at night, without a graduate nurse immediately at hand. Despite the possibility of such questionable practices, all else being equal, a hospital that has a nursing school or is approved for training by the AMA Council on Medical Education is preferable to one without such a program.

3. WHO "OWNS" THE HOSPITAL? The third major question to ask about a hospital concerns its ownership: Is it a voluntary, nonprofit, community hospital? Or is it a privately owned, pro-

prietary hospital? Or is it a third type, sponsored by the municipal, county, state, or federal government? (In some cases, patients in a government-sponsored hospital belong to a special category — service personnel and their dependents, veterans, members of Congress, etc.; these special hospitals are not considered in this chapter.)

Although the voluntary and proprietary hospitals generally tend to follow different patterns, the relationship between the quality of medical care in a hospital and its type of ownership is less direct than is the case with accreditation or teaching services. But in the judgment of CU's medical consultants, the voluntary hospital, when one has a choice, is to be preferred as a possible lead to a family doctor, and — with certain exceptions — by a prospective patient as well.

On the whole, government-supported hospitals also offer good medical facilities and competent staff. In those instances in which government-sponsored hospitals are affiliated with top-rated medical schools, the facilities and the staff may be superb. However, these institutions may fall behind voluntary hospitals in such matters as luxury accommodations and the number of private rooms.

By far the largest category of general hospitals, voluntary institutions number 3,339, and 2,800 of these are accredited by the JCAH. State-supported hospitals and those operated by units of local government total 1,761, with 1,087 accredited. Of the 775 proprietary hospitals, 517 have JCAH accreditation.

The voluntary hospital is a nonprofit community institution, functioning under religious or other voluntary auspices. The organizational structure of a voluntary nonprofit hospital, ideally, is designed to protect the patient in every possible way. Ultimate responsibility for all that transpires in such a hospital rests with its board of trustees, generally selected from among the community's business and professional people, who serve without pay. Few hospitals have as yet made provision for adequate consumer representation on hospital boards.

To manage the hospital, the trustees appoint a paid administrator — increasingly, in recent years, someone specially trained in the field of hospital administration, rather than a physician. The board generally does not invade the prerogatives of the medical staff. But when doctors disagree with hospital policy, as sometimes happens, the views of the board, acting through the administrator, generally prevail.

The proprietary hospitals are, in effect, commercial establishments, offering a special service to the public. The basic objectives of such institutions are less clear-cut and less open to generalization. They are, of course, intended to help sick people. They are also profit-making institutions, but the degree of their dedication to profit varies markedly. Some proprietary hospitals are set up by doctors in areas remote from a community hospital solely to provide a place to treat patients; if the hospital meets expenses, the owners are satisfied. Others may be strictly business propositions. It must be said, of course, that even a high degree of dedication to profit does not preclude high-quality medical care, any more than the nonprofit motive of community or voluntary hospitals assures good care.

Like the voluntary and proprietary hospitals, those sponsored by state and local governments vary widely in quality. The category of tax-supported institutions includes some very large hospitals — such as Bellevue in New York City — as well as some much smaller ones. All such institutions may sometimes be compelled to curtail services when budget allocations are cut. Publicly funded hospitals share a distinctive mission — they provide medical services for the indigent. Of course, any sick person, regardless of need, may be admitted to such hospitals. The nonindigent patient is usually billed according to standard rates.

As far as internal workings are concerned, one important factor differentiates the three types of hospitals. In the best of the voluntary hospitals, there are strict provisions for inspection, evaluation, and control of the medical activities of affiliated doctors. Government-sponsored institutions also tend to have rigid standards. On the whole, proprietary institutions are the least thorough. For example, in proprietary hospitals there are apt to be fewer restrictions on the scope of surgery performed by general practitioners. This means that in these hospitals it may be easier for physicians to perform operations they are not qualified to perform.

Although there are notable exceptions, proprietary hospitals tend to concentrate on the type of illness that can be treated relatively simply, without elaborate equipment or a highly specialized technical staff. They do surgical operations that generally call for a minimum of operating-room personnel and equipment — appendectomies, tonsillectomies, and voluntary abortions, for example. Rarely do proprietary hospitals go in for such complex — and expensive — procedures as open-heart surgery. Statistically, proprietary hospitals have less than their proportional share of blood banks, electroencephalographic services, medical libraries, postoperative recovery rooms, radioactive-isotope departments, and therapeutic X-ray services.

The lack of some equipment and services may make a proprietary hospital a poor place to be if you have a serious, complicated illness. But for certain kinds of hospitalization — such as one requiring routine obstetric care or one calling chiefly for bed rest, traction, and analgesics because of an acute, severe, low-back disorder — a patient may do just as well medically, and perhaps even better financially, in a JCAH-accredited proprietary hospital. These hospitals may have a lower per-diem charge than comparable nonprofit hospitals as a result of reduced operating costs. Despite the hope for profit, and need to pay taxes (from which voluntary hospitals are exempt), proprietary hospitals, by offering fewer medical services, can sometimes effect a savings in capital expenditure and staff expenses.

Attractive surroundings — a recently painted interior, modern fixtures, and the like — can be reassuring and desirable in a hospital. But it is well to remember that the real worth of a hospital lies in the capabilities of its attending staff and the adequacy and competency of such basic ancillary services as the pathology department, the chemistry laboratory, and the radiology section. Your physician will make a diagnosis and formulate therapy on the basis of reports from these areas. The reliability of such reports determines the real value of a hospital.

These three major guides to choosing a hospital — accreditation, teaching services, and ownership status — may prove inadequate or irrelevant in some communities. There may be only one hospital in the area, and therefore no choice. Or perhaps the only hospitals available are small, nonaccredited, proprietary institutions. In such areas, the readers of this book might inquire into the possibility of sparking a drive for a community nonprofit hospital. Such a venture, however, takes considerable community effort and substantial sums of philanthropic money (which can sometimes be supplemented, so far as construction expenses are concerned, by government funds). In some areas there may be too small a population to sustain a hospital, too little public demand for such a project, or so little available in the way of contributions from corporations or wealthy citizens that a voluntary hospital cannot be maintained.

One way to improve the quality of hospital care in some areas is to link groups of voluntary nonprofit hospitals into a regional association. Perhaps the best known of these is New England's Bingham Associates Fund, whose pioneering program, initiated about forty years ago, demonstrated how the medical knowledge and the expensive facilities of a great urban medical center could be brought to physicians and their patients in the smaller, less well-equipped hospitals typical of rural and sparsely settled areas.

The hub of the Bingham program was the Tufts–New England Medical Center, of which the Tufts University School of Medicine and the Bingham Associates Fund, both in Boston, were units. Reaching out to fifty-six hospitals in Maine and Massachusetts, the system provided for the transmission of medical data and specimens from the small institutions to referral centers, and the return of analyses, diagnoses, and expert opinions to the outlying hospitals. Today, this analytic and diag-

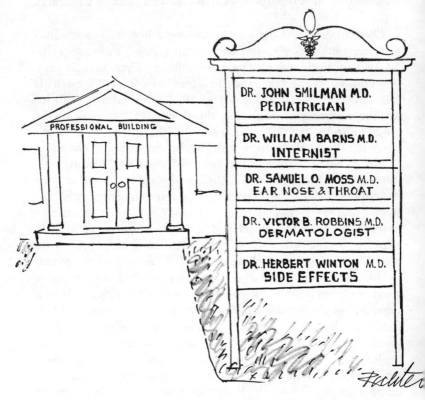

PROFESSIONAL BUILDING

DR. JOHN SMILMAN M.D.
PEDIATRICIAN

DR. WILLIAM BARNS M.D.
INTERNIST

DR. SAMUEL O. MOSS M.D.
EAR NOSE & THROAT

DR. VICTOR B. ROBBINS M.D.
DERMATOLOGIST

DR. HERBERT WINTON M.D.
SIDE EFFECTS

Drawing by Richter; © 1973 The New Yorker Magazine, Inc.

nostic work for the small outlying hospitals has been taken over by well-equipped regional hospitals in such Maine cities as Portland, Lewiston, and Waterville — with Tufts serving primarily as a communications center for the exchange of information.

If you lack such a setup or have no good hospital in your area, you would do well to ask your doctor about any working arrangements with a more distant good hospital. If someone in your family is seriously ill, the cost of transportation to such a place may be money well spent.

Even after you have made sure that your hospital is a good one, it is well to ask, whenever your doctor suggests that you or a member of your family enter the hospital, whether there is definite need for special services that cannot be provided at the doctor's office or at home. This is especially important for children and elderly people on whom removal to a hospital can impose serious emotional stresses. There are good reasons for staying out of a hospital unless you have to go there. For one thing, there is the expense. Unnecessary or prolonged hospitalizations eventually cause a rise in hospital insurance premiums. Nearly all hospitals have chronic staff shortages, which means that personal attention might be less than what the family could supply at home. Nearly all hospitals today are potential sources of infection; for example, the widespread use of antibiotics has encouraged the development of resistant strains of "staph" germs (see Chapter 28). If you really need to be in a hospital, however, these considerations should not deter you.

Glossary

This list of medical terms is selected from the pages of THE MEDI-CINE SHOW. Words and phrases defined here include those occurring in more than one chapter, those indispensable to understanding the material in a chapter, and those that may help clarify some of the definitions themselves. This last criterion is reflected in the frequent use of **bold face** as a guide to other terms in the glossary.

Not listed in the glossary are the names of drugs (over-the-counter and prescription), the names of most diseases, and words adequately defined in the book. Although the definitions are intended to ease reading of THE MEDICINE SHOW, they should also be of help in understanding other references to medical matters.

ABORT (a disease). To nip an ailment in the bud, when it has just begun to cause **symptoms.**

ABSORPTION. A process by which **drugs** and foods pass through a barrier, such as the intestinal wall or the skin, into the bloodstream.

ACID. A broad category of chemical substances, marked among other things by sour taste and a propensity to react with alkaline substances (bases) to form salts. Most bodily functions depend upon the maintenance of a balance between acids and bases in cells, blood, and other body fluids. (See also **acidification, buffered, neutralizing capacity.**)

ACIDIFICATION (urinary). In a healthy body, **acids** and bases are kept in balance by the excretion of acid in the urine. Certain **drugs** such as ascorbic acid (vitamin C) may increase the concentration of acid in the urine. The ability of the kidneys to excrete acid is impaired by certain diseases.

ACTINIC KERATOSIS. A horny growth on the skin resulting from longstanding exposure to the sun's actinic (ultraviolet) rays.

ACUTE. Describing an illness that comes on suddenly with strong sharp **symptoms** (such illnesses are usually of short duration), or any disease that needs urgent medical attention. (See also **chronic.**)

ADDICTIVE. Describing the property of certain **drugs,** such as **narcotics,** alcohol, and **barbiturates,** that leads to compulsive use by some people. Addiction generally manifests itself in three ways: tolerance to the drug develops so that the user no longer obtains the effect achieved with earlier dosage; physical withdrawal symptoms, sometimes even life-threatening, occur for a time if use of the addictive drug is curtailed; and recurrent craving for the drug is experienced even long after recovery from withdrawal symptoms.

ADRENAL GLANDS. A pair of **endocrine** glands, one perched atop each kidney. Among the major products of the adrenal glands' outer or **cortical** layer are the **corticosteroids,** notably **cortisone** and hydrocortisone. The inner core or medulla produces **adrenaline.**

ADRENALINE. A **hormone** secreted by the inner core or medulla of the **adrenal glands.** It acts on diverse organs and systems of the body to prepare one for "fight or flight," or other stressful situations. It is also available as the drug epinephrine (Adrenalin).

ALLERGEN. An **antigen** that causes an **allergy.**

ALLERGY. A person's abnormal reaction to a substance (called an **allergen**). It results from the body's immune mechanism being overwhelmed. **Symptoms** may include runny nose, red and itchy eyes, skin rash, wheezing, or sneezing. These symptoms are usually caused by the release of histamine. (See also **antihistamine, desensitization.**)

AMINO ACIDS. Basic chemical units into which food proteins are broken down during digestion, and from which body proteins are built up in various cells and organs, such as the liver.

ANALGESIC. A **drug**, such as aspirin or codeine, taken for relief of pain.

ANALOGUE. A chemical **compound** similar in structure to another chemical compound and having the same effect on body processes.

ANATOMIC. Having to do with the shape, structure, and relative position of the body's various parts, as distinct from their function (physiology) or malfunction (**pathology**).

ANEMIA. A reduction in the number of red blood cells whose function it is to distribute oxygen to all parts of the body. Anemic blood looks "washed out" — and that's how the patient feels.

ANESTHETIC. A **drug** used to deaden pain or to cause loss of consciousness. A local anesthetic dulls sensation at a specific spot or over a small portion of the body; a general anesthetic banishes pain by bringing on a deep artificial sleep; a **topical** anesthetic works just over the area of skin to which it is applied.

ANOREXIA. A **pathological** loss of appetite; aversion to food.

ANTACID. Short for antiacid — an alkaline **compound** that **neutralizes acid**, especially in the stomach.

ANTIBIOTIC. A substance that can kill harmful **microorganisms** in the body, or else keep them from multiplying until the body's own defenses can destroy them. Broad-spectrum antibiotics attack a wide range of germs; narrow-spectrum ones zero in on specific types. Unlike **antiseptics**, antibiotics are made by living organisms — **fungi** — from which they are extracted and refined for **pharmacological** use.

ANTIBODY. A protein substance produced by certain **white blood cells** in the body in response to injection, ingestion, or inhalation of an **antigen.** The production of an antibody can be beneficial, as in the case of immunization. (See also **immunological response, vaccine.**)

ANTICOAGULANT. A **drug** used to retard the **clotting** of blood. Typical anticoagulants are heparin (Meparin, Panheprin) and warfarin (Athrombin-K, Coumadin, Panwarfin).

ANTIGEN. A substance, alien to the body and usually a protein, which triggers the formation of an **antibody.**

ANTIHISTAMINE. A **drug** used to treat an **allergy** by counteracting the effects of histamine, a chemical manufactured by certain cells in the body.

ANTIHYPERTENSIVE. A drug taken by a person with **hypertension** to lower blood pressure and keep it lowered.

ANTIPRURITIC. A medication used to relieve itching. There are **topical** antipruritics, such as calamine lotion; others are taken internally.

ANTIPYRETIC. A **drug,** such as aspirin or acetaminophen, that lowers fever.

ANTISEPTIC. A chemical substance that destroys **microorganisms** on the skin, or curtails their multiplication. (See also **antibiotic, germicidal.**)

ASSAY. To analyze and quantify a substance.

ASTRINGENT. A substance that makes blood vessels or other tissues "pucker up" or contract. Alum, the material in styptic pencils, is a typical astringent used to stop small cuts from bleeding.

ASYMPTOMATIC. Without **symptoms**; signifying that an **infection** or disease is in a latent stage, is in **remission,** or simply is cured.

ATONIC. Flaccid, lacking **tone.** When a nerve is injured, the muscle supplied by that nerve becomes atonic. When intestinal muscles are atonic, **peristalsis** is inadequate and constipation results.

ATROPHY. A wasting or withering away of a part of the body from lack of use or from disruption of nerve supply or blood flow to that part of the body.

BACTERIA. General name for a vast variety of **microorganisms,** including beneficial as well as harmful types. "Good" bacteria make yogurt, aid digestion, and help to nourish growing plants. "Bad" or disease-producing bacteria cause all manner of **infectious** diseases.

BACTERIAL RESISTANCE. When a person acquires **immunity** against a strain of **bacteria,** that's good. But when the bacteria develop immunity of their own against an **antibiotic,** that's **resistance** — and that's bad.

BARBITURATE. A type of **drug** used in small doses as a **sedative,** and in larger doses as a **hypnotic.** Barbiturates may be **addictive.**

BELLADONNA ALKALOIDS. A mixture of plant derivatives including atropine, scopolamine, and related chemicals. As a group, the belladonna alkaloids work against the **parasympathetic nervous system**. One of their actions is to dry secretions of the **mucous membranes** in the mouth, nose, and stomach.

BIOCHEMICAL. Having to do with the nit-and-grit chemical composition of the body as well as its **metabolism**, rather than its **anatomy** or physiology.

BLIND TRIAL. A **controlled trial** of a **drug** in which the patients do not know whether they are being given the real thing or a **placebo** — but their doctors know. (See also **double-blind trial**.)

BONE MARROW FAILURE. Marrow, the soft pith or filling inside bones, manufactures the blood's red cells (which deliver oxygen throughout the body), white cells (which fight **infection**), and platelets (which help **clotting**). Certain **drugs,** as well as radiation, damage marrow so it cannot produce these cells; the phenomenon that results is known as bone marrow failure. Bone marrow failure may be partial, affecting only one type of blood cell rather than all three.

BRONCHI. Plural of bronchus; subdivisions of the trachea (windpipe) which further subdivide into bronchioles (narrower and narrower air tubes) descending deep into the lungs. Bronchitis is the name for **inflammation** of the bronchi.

BUFFERED. Describing therapeutic preparations to which antacids have been added. In the case of aspirin, buffering ostensibly protects the stomach against the corrosive effect of the aspirin.

CAPILLARY. The very finest subdivision of the body's network of blood vessels, the capillary is a microscopic blood vessel, much finer than a hair, with ultrathin walls, through which the blood gives up its oxygen to the body's tissues.

CARRIER. In **drugs** and cosmetics, the (relatively) **inert** substance in which the active ingredient is dissolved, mixed, or **suspended** for ease of administration.

CENTRAL NERVOUS SYSTEM. Consists of the brain and the spinal cord. The central nervous system controls mental activity plus voluntary — willed — muscular activity. It also coordinates the

parasympathetic and **sympathetic nervous systems,** which command the body's involuntary functions.

CHEMICAL CAUTERIZATION. A burning away of unwanted living tissue (warts, for example) by means of caustic **compounds,** such as strong **acids** or alkalies.

CHEMOTHERAPY. Treatment of disease (**therapy**) by medication with chemical **compounds.** Synonym: **drug** therapy.

CHROMOSOMES. The thousands of genes that carry hereditary messages from parents to offspring are strung on forty-six microscopic "necklaces" called chromosomes. The chromosomes are tightly coiled inside most body cells, including sperm and ova. These strings of genetic beads can be broken and partly lost or wrongly restrung by certain chemicals, **infectious** agents, radiation, and other factors − thus causing birth defects.

CHRONIC. Describing a disease of long duration or one that is recurrent. (See also **acute.**)

CLINICAL. Having to do with the medical care of ill people, and treatment of their signs and **symptoms,** as distinct from experimentation with laboratory animals. Thus a clinical trial involves trying new **therapy** on human subjects.

CLINICIAN. A practicing physician. Besides treating sick people, the clinician may (or may not) teach medicine and take part in medical research.

CLOTTING MECHANISM. The body's self-sealing system. When blood is shed, a complex series of **biochemical** reactions starts. The process ends with the manufacture of a tough substance called fibrin, which closes the wound and stops the bleeding. Certain **anticoagulants,** such as heparin (Meparin, Panheprin) and warfarin (Athrombin-K, Coumadin, Panwarfin), can disrupt this clotting or **coagulation** mechanism. The clotting mechanism is lacking in people afflicted with clotting factor deficiencies such as hemophilia.

COAGULATION. A synonym for **clotting.**

COMPOUND. In medical parlance, a preparation formed by combining several ingredients according to a formula. In chemical terms, a uniform substance formed by the stable combination of two or more chemical elements, as distinct from a mere mixture. (See also **molecular structure.**)

CONGESTION. The disruption of function in certain parts of the body by swelling of the lining tissues and by partial obliteration of the normal channels of blood flow or air flow. For instance, in **congestive heart failure,** congestion of the lungs occurs, making breathing arduous. Nasal congestion means swelling of the **mucous membranes** of the nose, making it difficult to breathe through the nose.

CONGESTIVE HEART FAILURE. A disorder characterized by swelling of the ankles and by shortness of breath. Congestive heart failure may follow a heart attack when the heart muscle has been severely damaged and thus can no longer function efficiently as a pump. Heart failure may also result from other forms of heart disease or from lung disease. (See also **coronary heart disease.**)

CONNECTIVE TISSUE. The "cement" of the body in which most cells are embedded. Connective tissue is made up for the most part of a material called collagen. Certain diseases, such as rheumatoid arthritis (see **rheumatology**), rheumatic fever, and lupus erythematosus, are disorders that primarily affect collagen.

CONTRAINDICATION. A reason not to use a given medication in a given situation; for example, many ordinarily beneficial **drugs** are contraindicated during pregnancy.

CONTROLLED TRIAL or STUDY. When a **drug** or other form of **therapy** is tried out **clinically,** to determine its efficacy, **toxicity, side effects,** indications, and **contraindications,** variable factors that could distort these results must be minimized. This is done by comparing the response of a trial group (patients who receive the new treatment) with that of a group of control subjects (patients who do not). The trial group and the control group are carefully matched for similarity in age, sex, and other relevant factors. (See also **blind trial, double-blind trial.**)

CORONARY HEART DISEASE. The name for the disorder that results from reduction in blood flow to the heart muscle due to narrowing of the coronary arteries by accumulation of fatty substances in the walls of the arteries. Activities that increase the heart rate can then cause transient chest pains (known as angina pectoris).

If a narrowed coronary artery becomes completely blocked by a blood clot (coronary thrombosis), the portion of the heart muscle supplied by that artery usually ceases to function. This is known as a heart attack — technically, myocardial infarction. (See also **congestive heart failure.**)

CORTICAL. Referring to the outer layer of certain organs. For instance, the cortical portion of the **adrenal glands** (adrenal cortex) secretes **corticosteroids.**

CORTICOSTEROID. A family of potent, versatile **hormones** originating mainly in the **adrenal glands,** used **therapeutically** (among other things) to treat **inflammatory** and **allergic** diseases. A corticosteroid can be produced naturally in the adrenal glands or synthesized in a laboratory.

CORTISONE. An **adrenal hormone,** one of the most important of the **corticosteroids,** used to treat **inflammatory** diseases.

CULTURE. A method of growing cells or **microorganisms** in the laboratory in order to identify them and to determine their **resistance** to **antibiotics.** The special food on which they are grown is the culture medium. (See also **in vitro, in vivo.**)

DECONGESTANT. A substance — usually a **vasoconstrictor** — that relieves nasal **congestion.**

DEGENERATIVE. Referring to changes in bodily function that reflect deterioration of certain cells or tissues, and the substances they secrete. For example, osteoarthritis is a degenerative joint disease.

DEMULCENT. A substance that soothes, softens, or protects a **mucous membrane** surface. An **emollient** does the same for skin.

DEPRESSANT. A **drug,** such as a **barbiturate** or alcohol, that acts on the **central nervous system** to diminish mental acuity and muscular activity.

DERMATITIS. An **inflammation** of the skin due to any of many causes, known and unknown. Thus contact dermatitis is a rash occurring as a reaction to some irritating chemical, textile, or other material touching or rubbing the skin. (See also **eczema.**)

DESENSITIZATION. A process by which **allergy** is reduced by periodic injection of gradually increasing amounts of the offending

allergen. A more accurate term for this process is hyposensitization because complete desensitization is rarely if ever achieved.

DETOXIFY. To remove or neutralize the harmful activity of a **toxin** in the body.

DIABETES MELLITUS. An all-too-familiar disorder of **metabolism,** in which the body cannot assimilate sugar for lack — or relative lack — of the hormone insulin. Popularly shortened to diabetes.

DIATHERMY. Deep heat **therapy,** generated by microwaves, aimed at muscles and joints. A microwave oven uses a similar principle.

DIURETIC. A **drug** that acts to eliminate fluid from the body by increasing the output of urine.

DOUBLE-BLIND TRIAL. A **controlled trial** of a **drug** in a **clinical** situation in which neither the recipients nor the experimenters (hence: double) know which patients are receiving the active substance, and which are being given a **placebo.** This dual ignorance minimizes subjective reactions to the drug being tested. (See also **blind trial.**)

DRUG. Medical meaning: Any chemical agent or medicinal substance (**compound,** preparation, remedy, etc.) used to promote health or to treat disease by causing a desired change within the body or on its surface. Popular meaning: Certain chemical compounds and plant substances that alter mood or mental or emotional state; some of these drugs are **addictive.**

DUODENAL ULCER. When the highly **acid** gastric juices of the stomach eat away at the wall of the duodenum (the first part of the small intestine below the stomach), the resulting raw sore is a duodenal ulcer. A duodenal ulcer may be painful and may bleed. If the ulcer heals with excessive scar tissue, an intestinal obstruction may result. (See also **peptic ulcer.**)

ECZEMA. A type of **dermatitis,** usually caused by an **allergy.**

ELECTROENCEPHALOGRAPHIC. Relating to the electroencephalograph (EEG) — a machine that helps a neurologist diagnose brain tumors, epilepsy, and other disorders by detecting abnormalities in the electrical waves emanating from different areas of the brain. Similar to the electrocardiograph (ECG) — a machine that helps a physician detect electrical impulses from the heart.

ELIXIR. A liquid form of the sugar-coated pill. A mixture of water, sweetener, scent, and alcohol, used as a **carrier** to make your medicine more pleasant to take.

EMOLLIENT. A substance — such as petrolatum or olive oil — that soothes, softens, or protects the skin surface. A **demulcent** does the same for **mucous membrane.**

ENDOCRINE SYSTEM. An interlocking directorate of glands whose **hormones** control bodily growth, sex characteristics, **metabolism,** and many other functions. The main endocrine glands are the **adrenals,** ovaries, pancreas, parathyroids, **pituitary,** testes, and thyroid.

ENZYMES. Proteins made by the body which act as catalysts for many **biochemical** reactions. Enzymes also break down food and other substances into simpler chemical **compounds** which can then be absorbed, **metabolized,** or otherwise used by the body. Enzymes are also used commercially; meat tenderizer, for instance, is an enzyme.

EUPHORIA. In medical terms, an exaggerated feeling of well-being or elation.

FOLIC ACID. A nutrient used by the **bone marrow** in the production of red blood cells.

FREE FATTY ACID. An organic **acid** "freed" from a more complex **compound** in the **metabolism** of body fat.

FUNCTIONAL DISEASE. A disorder due to faulty working of one or more otherwise healthy organs or parts of the body. As opposed to **organic disease.**

FUNGUS. A parasitic **microorganism,** best known as the itchy villain in athlete's foot. The category also includes some medically more important types which infect internal organs and can even cause death. Some fungi, though, are beneficial — such as the molds that produce **antibiotics,** and the yeast that makes bread rise.

GASTROINTESTINAL. Having to do with the digestive tract including the esophagus, stomach, small intestine, large intestine, and rectum. Abbreviated "GI," as in GI series which is an X-ray visualization of the upper part of the gastrointestinal tract taken after the patient swallows a radiopaque substance such as barium.

GEL. A substance of jellylike consistency.

GENERIC. Describing the name given to a **drug** by the United States Adopted Names Council (see Chapter 30), as distinct from the registered brand name a pharmaceutical company gives to its version of the same preparation.

GERMICIDAL. Referring to chemical agents, lethal to germs, which are generally used as **topical** applications. Describes the action of certain **antiseptics**. (See also **microorganisms**.)

GLAUCOMA. A serious eye disease caused by build-up of fluid pressure inside the eyeball. Simple or **chronic** glaucoma usually comes on gradually as part of the **degenerative** aging process; if untreated, it usually destroys the optic nerve, causing blindness. Closed-angle (also known as narrow-angle) or **acute** glaucoma has a sudden severe onset due to narrowing of the eyeball's natural drainage channels. Acute glaucoma is accompanied by severe pain; if untreated, it can lead to irreparable damage.

GRAIN. The apothecary's traditional unit of weight – approximately 65/1,000 of a **gram**. It is still used by doctors in prescribing – and by pharmacists in compounding – pills, powders, and potions. (See also **milligram**.)

GRAM. A unit of weight in the metric system, often used to measure **drugs** and food. Approximately 28 grams are equal to 1 ounce; 1/1,000 of a gram is a **milligram**. (See also **grain**.)

GRAM-NEGATIVE and -POSITIVE. **Bacteria** are of two varieties: Gram-positive bacteria are visible under the microscope when dyed by a certain technique – Gram's stain; Gram-negative bacteria fail to hold the color. (Named after Hans Gram, a Danish bacteriologist, not after the **gram** unit of weight.)

GRANULOMAS. Microscopic **lesions** composed of whorls of **inflammatory** tissue. Granuolmas are present in such diseases as **sarcoidosis**, tuberculosis, and certain **fungal infections**.

HALLUCINOGEN. A **drug** that may in some individuals cause hallucinations, either auditory or visual.

HALOGENS. A group of related chemical elements – chlorine, iodine, bromine, and fluorine. They combine readily with hydrogen to form **acids**, and with metals to form salts.

HEMOLYTIC. Referring to the process of hemolysis by which the membrane surrounding a red blood cell breaks. This may be caused by a defect in the red cell membrane itself (as in sickle cell **anemia**) or by an **antibody** that clings to and damages the membrane.

HEMORRHAGE. Excessive loss of blood from the body or into its inner cavities through cut or torn veins, arteries, or **capillaries**.

HORMONE. A chemical substance made in an **endocrine** gland and secreted into the bloodstream. The hormone then acts on some distant target within the body.

HOST. (1) An organism (especially a human being) in and on which an invading microorganism thrives. (2) An individual who receives a donor transplant organ.

HOUSE STAFF. Medical doctors enrolled in a hospital training program; popularly referred to as interns and residents.

HYPER-. A prefix meaning more than normal.

HYPERTENSION. A disorder that is characterized by increased blood pressure. If undetected or untreated, hypertension may eventually affect the functioning of the brain, eyes, heart, and kidneys.

HYPNOTIC. A **drug** that induces sleep. Some hypnotics, in smaller dosage, are used as daytime **sedatives**.

HYPO-. A prefix meaning less than normal.

IDIOPATHIC. A medical term used to describe a disease of unknown cause or origin.

IMMUNE MECHANISM. See **immunological response**.

IMMUNITY. **Resistance** to a specific **infection**. (See also **vaccine**.)

IMMUNOLOGICAL RESPONSE. The production of specific proteins called **antibodies** by certain **white blood cells** in response to stimulation by specific **antigens** (e.g., **bacteria**, **viruses**, pollens). The antibodies resist in varying degrees invasion of the body by these **microorganisms** and other alien substances. Transfused blood of the wrong type or an organ transplanted from another body can also induce this response.

INCUBATE. To facilitate growth or multiplication of cells or germs in a **culture** medium (**in vitro**) to the point where they can be identified, or **in vivo** to the point where they cause **symptoms.**

INERT. Without physiological action or effect, as a **placebo.**

INFECTION. (1) Invasion of the body, or one of its parts, by a harmful **microorganism.** (2) The disease thus caused.

INFLAMMATION. The body's four-alarm response to injury or infection: (1) pain, (2) heat, (3) reddening, and (4) swelling. These local reactions signify that the body is rallying its forces to limit and repair the damage. Inflammation is thus not the same as **infection,** although the latter often triggers inflammation.

IN VITRO. Literally, "in glass" – a medical or biological event that takes place outside the human body in the laboratory. As opposed to **in vivo.** (See also **culture, incubate.**)

IN VIVO. Literally, "in life" – a medical or biological event that takes place in a living human or animal. As opposed to **in vitro.** (See also **culture, incubate.**)

IODIDE. Iodide-containing salts such as sodium iodide or potassium iodide. Iodide that is ingested in food or medication is avidly picked up by the thyroid gland where it is used for the manufacture of thyroid **hormones.** Radioactive iodide is often used to diagnose and treat certain thyroid diseases. (See also **radioactive isotope.**)

IRREVERSIBLE. A medical term for incurable. A one-way process of deterioration that may be arrested, perhaps, but never corrected.

-ITIS. A suffix meaning **inflammation** of, as in appendicitis.

LESION. Any damaged site or local **pathological** condition in skin or internal tissue, caused by disease, **degeneration,** or injury.

MEMBRANE. See **mucous membrane.**

METABOLISM. The **biochemical** processes by which food and oxygen are used by the body to provide the energy that is necessary for the proper functioning of body organs and tissues.

MICROORGANISMS. Living creatures too small to be seen with the naked eye. **Pathological** microorganisms, which cause **infections** in larger forms of life, are known colloquially as germs. They include **viruses, bacteria,** and **fungi.**

MILLIGRAM. 1/1,000 of a gram; the metric unit of weight in

which **drug** dosages are measured. (See also **grain, gram.**)

MOLECULAR STRUCTURE. The architecture of a **compound**. By making small changes in the molecular structure of a **drug, analogues** are produced and the **pharmacological** effects of the original substance may be altered.

MUCOUS MEMBRANE. The body's "inside skin" — extremely thin, soft layers of cells that line the surface of certain body tracts such as the respiratory tract and the gastrointestinal tract.

MUCUS. A slimy, colorless substance secreted by the **mucous** cells of the intestines and respiratory tract.

NARCOTIC. A natural or synthetic **addictive drug** used medically to relieve pain or to produce sleep by **depressing** the **central nervous system.** Examples are codeine, meperidine, and morphine.

NEPHROLOGY. A branch of medical science dealing with the kidney — its structure, functions, and diseases.

NEUTRALIZING CAPACITY. The ability of an alkali to offset acidity. (See also **antacid.**)

NF. Refers to a **drug** compounded according to the *National Formulary*, a semiofficial directory of drug standards and specifications, issued every five years by the American Pharmaceutical Association. (See also **USP.**)

NODULAR THYROID. A thyroid gland that has one or more lumps that can be felt through the skin of the neck. A nodular thyroid requires evaluation by a physician.

NOSTRUM. A "remedy" for which extravagant, scientifically unsupported therapeutic claims are often made; a **patent medicine.**

OCCLUSION. In general, the closing or blocking of a blood vessel or some other passageway or orifice in the body. In dentistry, the manner in which upper and lower teeth meet when the jaws shut; the "bite."

ONCOLOGY. A branch of medical science dealing with tumors (particularly cancers) — their origin, nature, growth, effects, and treatment.

ORGANIC DISEASE. A disorder due to **anatomic** changes in a body organ that interfere with an organ's ability to do its job. As opposed to **functional disease** of a structurally intact organ. For example, rectal cancer, an organic disease, may cause constipation. Constipation triggered by a family crisis would be a functional type of bowel disorder.

OVER-THE-COUNTER (OTC) DRUG. A drug that the Food and Drug Administration (FDA) accepts as safe for self-medication. According to the FDA, an OTC drug can be used by consumers for disorders they diagnose themselves and treat by following the directions on the label without advice from a physician. As opposed to **prescription drug.**

PARASYMPATHETIC NERVOUS SYSTEM. A network of nerves that controls such involuntary, unconscious, automatic bodily reactions as dilatation of certain blood vessels, slowdown in heartbeat, narrowing of pupils, salivation, and increased nasal secretion. The **sympathetic nervous system** generally has opposite effects.

PATENT MEDICINE. An **over-the-counter** preparation whose formula is usually a trade secret, and for which unproven **therapeutic** benefits are often claimed; a **nostrum.**

PATHOLOGICAL. Describing an abnormality usually caused by disease.

PEPTIC ULCER. A raw, sore eroded area on the wall of the stomach or **duodenum.** When the wall of the stomach or duodenum is eaten all the way through, the **lesion** is called a **perforation.** If a blood vessel is eroded in the process, bleeding occurs — hence the familiar bleeding ulcer.

PERFORATION (of ulcer). See **peptic ulcer.**

PERINATAL. Referring to the time period from birth to approximately one month afterward.

PERISTALSIS. Synchronized, sequential contractions of special muscles in the **gastrointestinal** tract that nudge and squeeze food through the esophagus and stomach to the intestine and rectum.

PHARMACOLOGICAL. Concerning the action — **therapeutic** or **toxic** or both — of a **drug** on or in the body; its **absorption, metabolism,** and excretion, as well as its effect on cells, tissues, organs, and bodily function.

PHOTOSENSITIVITY REACTION. A heightened sensitivity of the skin to the rays of the sun, caused by certain oral medications and cosmetics.

PITUITARY. An **endocrine** gland located at the base of the brain: the body's main "command module." Its **hormones** direct the activities of the **adrenal glands,** ovaries, testes, and thyroid, and also govern such key processes as growth and **metabolism.**

PLACEBO. A medically **inert** substance formulated to mimic — in color and form — an active substance; used in testing the efficacy of a **drug.** The patients in a **blind trial** (and their doctors as well in a **double-blind trial**) do not know who receives the active substance, or who the dummy one. In **clinical** studies as many as 40 percent of the subjects respond favorably to a placebo.

PRESCRIPTION DRUG. A drug available only by doctor's prescription; too potent or dangerous or **addictive** to be sold to all comers. (See also **over-the-counter drug.**)

PSYCHOSIS. One of a group of serious mental or emotional disorders, notably **schizophrenia** and manic-depressive psychosis, which may impair mental functioning sufficiently to interfere with capacity to meet the ordinary demands of life.

PSYCHOSOMATIC. Referring to a group of physical ailments that are known to be caused by emotional factors. These are not imagined illnesses, but conditions in which actual evidence of physical disease can be documented. For example, some bowel disorders, **bronchial** asthma, and **peptic ulcer** are considered psychosomatic illnesses.

PSYCHOTHERAPEUTIC DRUG. A chemical **compound** that is prescribed by a physician in the treatment of mental or emotional disorders.

PSYCHOTHERAPY. The treatment of mental or emotional disorders primarily by interaction between therapist and patient, or therapist and a group of patients, or interaction among patients without a therapist. Its methods include suggestion, persuasion, hypnosis, dream analysis, free-association analysis, and the like.

PULMONARY. Having to do with the lungs.

RADIOACTIVE ISOTOPE. A kind of chemical element, either natural or man-made in a nuclear reactor, that emits energy in the form of radiation that can be detected by instruments. The isotope of a particular element can mimic its natural counterpart in body **metabolism.** As a result, certain chemical **compounds** "tagged" with the radioactive isotope can be swallowed or injected and followed through the body by a radiation detector, making possible many kinds of diagnostic tests. Large doses of radioactive isotopes may be used **therapeutically.**

REBOUND EFFECT. An intense flare-up of **symptoms** related to the use of medication which occurs when the medication is suddenly withdrawn or its effects wear off. The rebound symptoms are generally more severe than those for which the medication was originally taken. In order to suppress these symptoms the patient may resort to more frequent use of the medication or increased dosage or both. The rebound effect most commonly occurs with the use of nose drops. It also occurs with abrupt discontinuance of corticosteroids and occasionally other oral medications.

REFLEX. An automatic, involuntary action of a muscle in response to nerve stimulation. An unconditioned reflex is one built into the nervous system of every normal human being (e.g., the knee-jerk reaction). A conditioned reflex is one that has been learned by experience (e.g., a dog drooling at the sound of a dinner bell).

REGIMEN. Just what the doctor orders; any **therapeutic** program or schedule for eating, sleeping, exercising, taking medicine, and so forth.

REMISSION. Temporary absence of signs and **symptoms** of a disease, usually an incurable one.

RESISTANT. **Immune** to or unaffected by. (See also **bacterial resistance.**)

RHEUMATIC. Having to do with rheumatism — sore, stiff, inflamed joints and muscles due to various causes, known and unknown.

RHEUMATOLOGY. The branch of medical science dealing with **rheumatic** diseases (such as rheumatoid arthritis and gout) or diseases of **connective tissue.**

SALICYLATES. A class of **compounds** (of which aspirin is the best known) used to relieve pain, reduce **inflammation**, and lower body temperature.

SARCOIDOSIS. A generalized disorder in which **granulomas** develop in various organs of the body, primarily the lungs, but also the liver, lymph nodes, and spleen. The cause of sarcoidosis is unknown. Severe cases are treated with a **corticosteroid**.

SCHIZOPHRENIA. One of a group of **psychoses**, in which the affected person undergoes personality changes marked by withdrawal and bizarre behavior. Hallucinations, delusions, and paranoia are not uncommon.

SCREENING TEST. A mass examination of a large group or population designed to detect a particular disease early enough to treat it with maximum effect.

SEDATIVE. A **drug** that exerts a calming or quieting effect on mental processes or nervous irritability. (See also **tranquilizer**.)

SENSITIZATION. Stimulation of the body's **immunological response** "memory" by a foreign substance, so that the next time the alien material makes contact — which may be even years later — **symptoms** of the **allergy** may appear.

SERUM FACTORS. In the serum (the liquid part of the blood) there are various types of **antibodies** which help the **white blood cells** to overwhelm infecting microorganisms. Serum factors may also be associated with certain diseases such as rheumatoid arthritis (see **rheumatology**) or thyroiditis.

SHOTGUN REMEDY. A medication combining two or more different **therapeutic drugs** in a single preparation, presumably based on the theory that if you use enough ingredients, one might work.

SIDE EFFECT. The cloud inside the silver lining. Every **drug**, along with its desired **pharmacological** action, causes other gratuitous consequences, ranging from incidental to downright **toxic**. Because these dividends — usually unwelcome — may be dose-related, proper **chemotherapy** must specify the exact quantity of **drugs** that offers the best trade-off between benefit and burden to the body.

SIGN. See **symptom**.

SMEAR. A sample of blood, **mucus**, pus, or other material from the body spread on a glass slide for staining and examination under a microscope.

SODIUM. One of the two chemical elements in table salt (the other is chlorine). In the body, sodium is one of the most important constitutents of blood and of other body fluids. People with **congestive heart failure** or **hypertension** may be advised to reduce sodium in their diet.

SPASM. Voluntary or involuntary contraction (clenching, tensing, or tightening up) of muscles.

SPHINCTER. A round muscle encircling an opening in the body; when it contracts, it is capable of closing the orifice.

SPUTUM. **Mucus**, sometimes mixed with pus, coughed up from the lungs and **bronchial** tubes. Synonym: phlegm.

STEROIDS. A family of organic **compounds**, or their **analogues**, of which the **corticosteroid hormones** secreted by the **adrenal glands** are a subdivision. Steroids perform a vital function in the process of **metabolism**.

SUBACUTE. Midway between **acute** and **chronic** in the course of a disease.

SUBCLINICAL. A stage of a disease or abnormality at which characteristic **symptoms** are lacking. A disease that remains subclinical may come and go without ever being diagnosed as a specific **clinical** disorder.

SUSPENSION. A uniform mixture of insoluble fine particles in water or some other liquid. Shake well before using!

SYMPATHETIC NERVOUS SYSTEM. A network of nerves that trigger certain involuntary or automatic bodily functions, such as constricting blood vessels, making hair stand on end, raising "gooseflesh" on the skin, widening the pupils, contracting most **sphincters**, and speeding up the heartbeat. These stimuli add up to the "startle reaction" by which the body mobilizes for "fight or flight" in the face of sudden danger or surprise. (See also **parasympathetic nervous system.**)

SYMPTOM. What the patient complains of — from bad breath to

palpitations to pain. A symptom is your body's signal to you that something is wrong (e.g., abdominal pain) and a clue to your doctor as to what its cause is likely to be. A sign, on the other hand, is what your doctor finds on examination (e.g., tenderness of the abdomen). One sign or symptom does not (usually) a **syndrome** make, but several signs and symptoms do.

SYMPTOMATIC RELIEF. The amelioration of **symptoms** of disease by such measures as the administration of medicine. For example, aspirin is commonly used for relief of pain, which is a symptom, rather than as treatment for the underlying cause of the pain.

SYNDROME. A set or constellation of **symptoms** or signs which together characterize or identify a specific disease or disorder.

SYSTEMIC. Referring to the body as a whole, rather than to one of its parts or organs.

THERAPEUTIC EQUIVALENT. A **drug** that can be substituted for another without loss of efficacy.

THERAPY. Any form of medical treatment.

TIMED-RELEASE. A form of medication in which the active **drug** is purportedly absorbed into the bloodstream gradually over an extended period. Actually, the release rate may be highly variable from person to person and dose to dose.

TOLERANCE. See **addictive.**

TONE. A steady state of "stretch" or tension in healthy muscles enabling them to be always ready to respond rapidly to stimuli. Certain diseases diminish this normal tonicity, rendering muscles **atonic.**

TOPICAL. Applied directly on the skin (or accessible **mucous membrane**) to treat a **lesion** at its local site, rather than administered **systemically** (i.e., throughout the body, by way of the bloodstream or digestive tract).

TOXIC. Poisonous: effect ranging from harmful to lethal, depending on the dose and the resistance of the individual. (See also **detoxify.**)

TRANQUILIZER. A **drug** used to relieve anxiety and to calm. Major tranquilizers are used to treat **psychoses;** minor tranquilizers are used to relieve **symptoms** of anxiety and, sometimes, to relieve emotional stress associated with **organic disease**. Because it is less likely to produce drowsiness, a tranquilizer may be preferable to a **sedative**, particularly for daytime use.

TROCHE. A pill or lozenge that is dissolved in the mouth.

TUMOR. An abnormal growth on or in the body, which serves no useful purpose. A tumor may be malignant (cancerous) or benign (noncancerous).

URETHRA. A narrow drainpipe (shorter in women than in men) through which the bladder voids urine. When the urethra is narrowed, as may happen with recurrent infection, it may have to be surgically stretched (dilated) to restore outflow.

UROLOGY. The branch of surgery dealing with the urinary tract — kidneys, ureters, bladder, **urethra** — plus (in males) the prostate gland and genitals.

USP. Refers to a **drug** compounded according to the *United States Pharmacopeia*, a semiofficial **pharmacological** directory of drug standards and specifications, issued every five years by a national committee of physicians, pharmacists, and academicians. (See also **NF.**)

VACCINE. A specially formulated mix of a weakened or killed **infection**-causing **bacterium** or **virus** introduced into the body so that the body through its immune mechanism will develop **antibodies** against the same bacterium or virus. These antibodies serve as protection against infection with the naturally occurring bacterium or virus.

VAPORIZER. A device for adding moisture or humidity to the air of a room. A cool-mist model does this by atomizing water into microdroplets. An electrolytic vaporizer boils water to steam up the atmosphere. A boiler-type vaporizer is also available.

VARICOSE VEINS. Abnormal veins that have become permanently stretched. There is an increased tendency for blood flow to slow down and for **clots** to form in these veins. Varicose veins usually occur in the legs and the anal region.

VASCULAR. Having to do with the blood's delivery system — arteries, veins, and **capillaries**.

VASOCONSTRICTOR. A chemical substance that narrows or shrinks the diameter of arteries and thereby reduces blood supply to an organ or tissue.

VIRUS. This smallest of all **microorganisms** causes a variety of viral infections, from fever blisters and German measles to polio. Some viruses are suspected of triggering certain cancers. A virus works havoc by invading a cell, disrupting its internal functioning, and distorting its reproduction mechanism.

WHITE BLOOD CELLS. Cells in the bloodstream which fight off **infection** by harmful **microorganisms.** One kind of white cell actually attacks **bacteria.** The other kind helps by making **antibodies.** Dead white cells and tissue, along with killed bacteria, collect as pus. (See also **serum factors.**)

WITHDRAWAL. See **addictive.**

Product index

373

General index